BENDING BUT NOT BREAKING

LIVING WITH EHLERS-DANLOS SYNDROME

DR. MOHAMMAD E. BARBATI

INTRODUCTION

When you hear the term "connective tissue disorders," you might not immediately think of conditions that can significantly impact one's quality of life. However, for individuals living with Ehlers-Danlos Syndrome (EDS), the reality of dealing with a connective tissue disorder is ever-present. In this book, we'll delve into the definition of EDS and provide an overview of connective tissue disorders to better understand the challenges faced by those living with these conditions.

DEFINITION

Ehlers-Danlos Syndrome: A Closer Look

Ehlers-Danlos Syndrome (EDS) is a group of inherited disorders that primarily affect the connective tissues in the body, which provide support, structure, and stability to our organs, joints, and skin. These connective tissues are composed of proteins such as collagen, which plays a vital role in maintaining the integrity and elasticity of various bodily structures.

Individuals with EDS often experience hypermobility of joints, skin that is easily bruised and hyper-elastic, and a tendency to develop scars easily. The severity of symptoms can vary greatly, with some individuals experiencing relatively mild manifestations, while others face life-threatening complications.

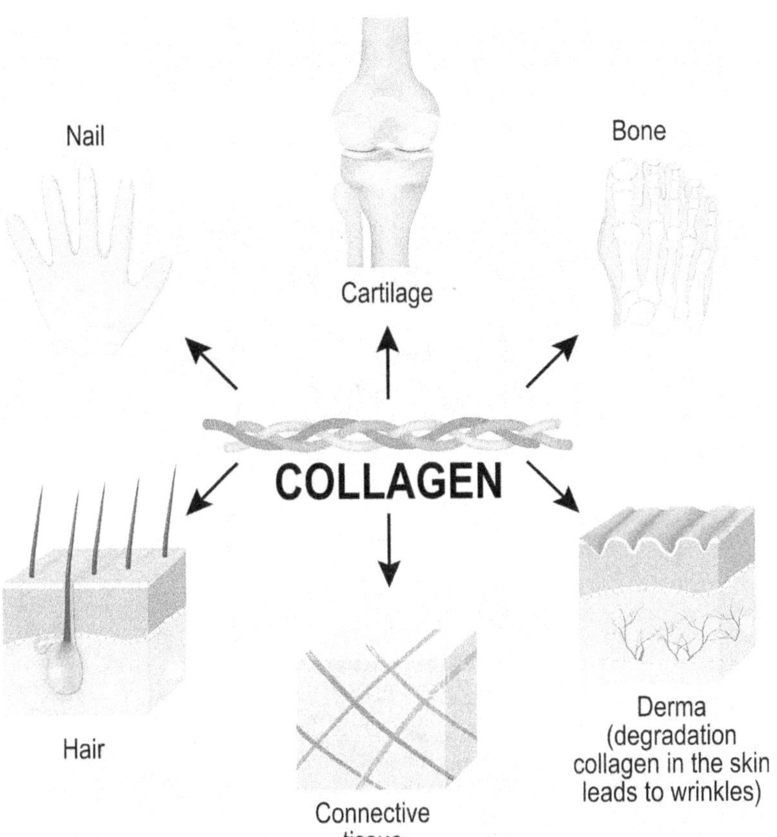
Nail
Cartilage
Bone
COLLAGEN
Hair
Connective
tissue
Derma
(degradation
collagen in the skin
leads to wrinkles)

OVERVIEW OF CONNECTIVE TISSUE DISORDERS

Connective Tissue Disorders: A Broad Landscape

Connective tissue disorders encompass a wide range of conditions that affect the body's connective tissues. These disorders can be inherited, such as EDS and Marfan Syndrome, or acquired due to factors like autoimmune diseases (e.g., lupus and rheumatoid arthritis) and environmental factors.

These conditions can impact various aspects of an individual's life, from joint pain and mobility issues to skin problems and even cardiovascular complications. Since connective tissues are found throughout the body, the manifestations of these disorders can vary drastically from one person to another.

Inherited Connective Tissue Disorders

In addition to EDS, other inherited connective tissue disorders include:

- **Marfan Syndrome:** A genetic disorder that affects the body's connective tissue, causing symptoms such as long limbs, scoliosis, and heart problems.
- **Osteogenesis Imperfecta:** A condition characterized by brittle bones that break easily, often caused by a genetic mutation affecting collagen production.
- **Stickler Syndrome:** A genetic disorder that can cause vision, hearing, and joint problems due to abnormal collagen production.

Acquired Connective Tissue Disorders

Some connective tissue disorders are acquired, meaning they develop due to factors other than genetics. Examples include:

- **Systemic Lupus Erythematosus:** An autoimmune disease where the immune system mistakenly attacks healthy tissue, leading to inflammation and damage to various body systems.
- **Rheumatoid Arthritis:** A chronic inflammatory disorder that affects the joints and can cause pain, swelling, and stiffness.
- **Scleroderma:** A group of rare diseases that cause the skin and connective tissues to harden and tighten.

By exploring the world of connective tissue disorders, we can better understand the challenges faced by those living with conditions like EDS. As research continues to advance, we hope to find better ways to diagnose, manage, and treat these disorders, improving the quality of life for those affected. If you found this information engaging and insightful, we encourage you to explore further and learn more about the fascinating world of connective tissue disorders.

CLASSIFICATION AND SUBTYPES

**A Mosaic of Symptoms:
The Many Faces of EDS**

EDS is a highly variable condition, with symptoms ranging from mild to severe, depending on the affected individual. Some of the most common manifestations include:

- **Skin** that is easily bruised, hyper-elastic, and prone to scarring
- Unstable joints that are prone to frequent dislocations and increased mobility beyond the normal range
- **Chronic pain** in muscles, joints, and bones
- **Blood vessels** that are easily damaged, leading to spontaneous bruising or, in severe cases, life-threatening complications

Given the wide spectrum of symptoms, it's essential to have a comprehensive classification system that can help healthcare professionals accurately diagnose and manage EDS.

The Evolution of EDS Classification: A Journey Through Time

The classification of EDS has evolved over time, with various attempts to organize the different subtypes according to their unique characteristics. Initially, EDS was classified based on Roman numerals, but this system was later replaced by a more descriptive approach that focused on the primary clinical features of each subtype.

As scientific understanding of EDS grew, so too did the need for an updated classification system. The latest EDS classification system, published in 2017, represents the most comprehensive and accurate classification to date, providing a solid foundation for future research and clinical care. This system is based on a combination of clinical, genetic, and molecular criteria, allowing for a more precise and thorough assessment of the different EDS subtypes.

The Underlying Genetics of EDS

At the heart of the EDS classification system lies the intricate world of genetics. The different EDS subtypes are caused by mutations in various genes, which in turn affect the structure, function, and production of specific proteins involved in connective tissue. By understanding the genetic basis of each subtype, researchers can develop targeted therapies and better management strategies that cater to the unique needs of those affected.

Remarkably, the EDS classification system is not set in stone. As our understanding of the disorder grows, new subtypes may be identified, and existing ones might be refined. This constantly evolving landscape highlights the importance of staying up-to-date with the latest research and developments.

CLASSICAL EDS

Classical EDS (cEDS) is characterized by a range of symptoms that primarily affect the skin and joints. Individuals with cEDS often experience:

- Hyper-elastic, fragile skin that is prone to bruising and tearing easily
- Atrophic scarring, where the skin forms thin, cigarette paper-like scars
- Joint hypermobility, which leads to an increased range of motion and a higher risk of joint dislocations and injuries
- Chronic pain in muscles, joints, and bones due to repeated injuries and strain on the connective tissue

While the symptoms of cEDS can be challenging to manage, understanding the underlying genetic basis of the condition can provide valuable insights for potential treatment options.

Unraveling the Genetic Code:
The Root Cause of cEDS

Classical EDS is caused by mutations in specific genes that are responsible for the production of collagen, a primary component of connective tissue. Collagen forms a network of fibers that provide strength and flexibility to our skin, joints, and other tissues. In cEDS, these collagen fibers are less robust, which leads to the characteristic symptoms of the condition.

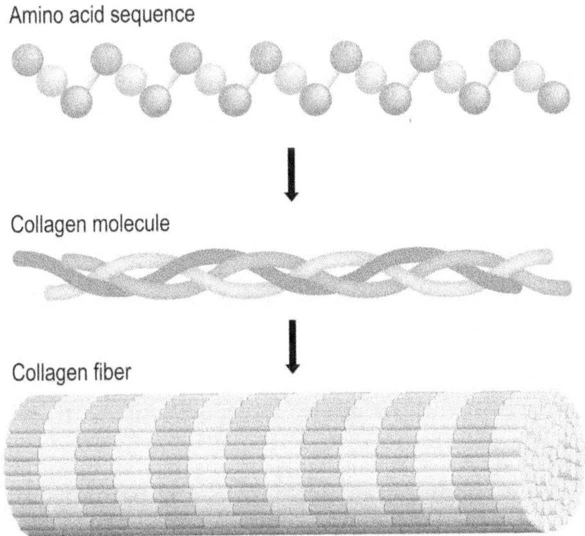

Molecular structure of collagen

CLASSICAL-LIKE EDS

Classical-like EDS (clEDS) is marked by a range of symptoms that primarily affect the skin and joints, with some overlap with other EDS subtypes. Individuals with clEDS often experience:

- Hyper-elastic, soft skin that can be easily bruised or damaged
- A lack of significant scarring, which distinguishes it from other EDS subtypes
- Joint hypermobility, leading to an increased range of motion and a higher risk of joint dislocations and injuries
- Chronic pain in muscles, joints, and bones due to repeated injuries and strain on the connective tissue

While clEDS symptoms can pose challenges for those affected, understanding the underlying genetic basis of the condition can offer valuable insights for potential treatment options.

Decoding the Genetic Puzzle: The Root Cause of Classical-like EDS

Classical-like EDS is caused by mutations in a specific gene that plays a crucial role in the formation of the extracellular matrix, a complex network of proteins and carbohydrates that provides support and structure to cells and tissues. In clEDS, the function of this gene is impaired, leading to alterations in the extracellular matrix and the characteristic symptoms of the condition.

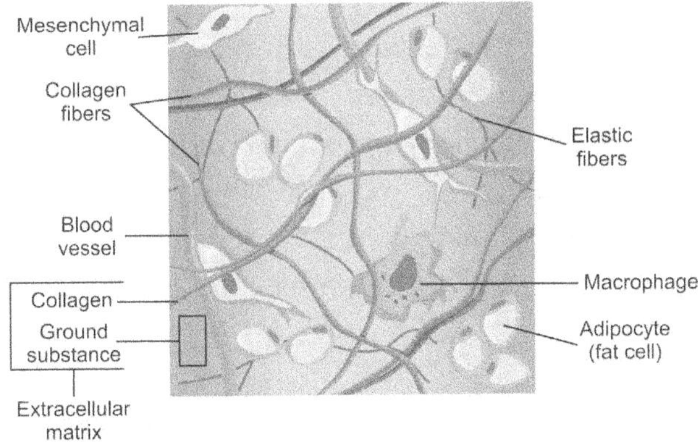

Connective tissue and the extracellular matrix

Genetic testing can be an essential tool in confirming the diagnosis of clEDS and pinpointing the specific gene mutations involved. This information is invaluable for healthcare professionals, as it allows them to provide targeted care and support to individuals with the condition.

CARDIAC-VALVULAR EDS

Cardiac-Valvular EDS, or cvEDS, is an uncommon form of EDS that predominantly affects the heart valves. This condition is characterized by a range of symptoms, including joint hypermobility, skin fragility, and, most notably, cardiac valvular abnormalities. The latter can manifest as valvular insufficiency or prolapse, which can lead to life-threatening complications if left untreated.

The Genetics Behind cvEDS: A Closer Look

Like other forms of EDS, cvEDS is an inherited condition passed down through families. More specifically, it is an autosomal recessive disorder, meaning that an individual must inherit two copies of the mutated gene—one from each parent—to develop the condition. The gene responsible for cvEDS is called COL1A2, which encodes the pro-alpha2(I) chain of type I collagen. Mutations in the COL1A2 gene result in the production of structurally abnormal collagen, which in turn causes the various symptoms associated with cvEDS.

Diagnosing Cardiac-Valvular EDS: Challenges and Solutions

Considering the rarity of cvEDS, diagnosing this condition can be challenging. Patients often present with a wide range of symptoms, some of which may overlap with other forms of EDS or unrelated disorders. As a result, healthcare professionals must rely on a combination of clinical observations, family history, and genetic testing to accurately diagnose cvEDS.

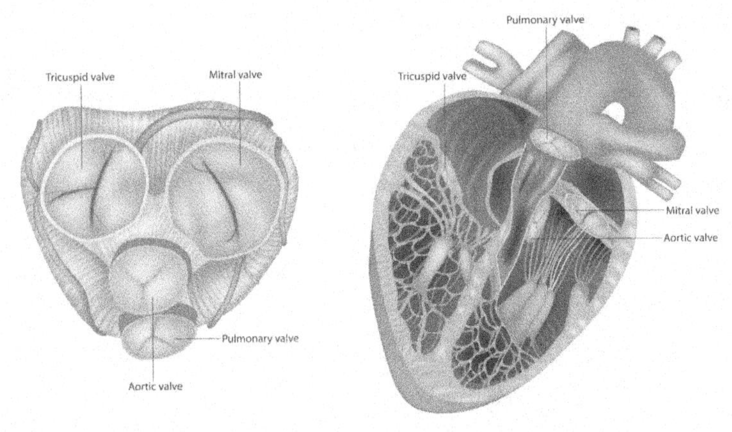

Structure of the Heart valves anatomy

VASCULAR EDS

Vascular EDS, or vEDS, is a rare form of EDS that primarily affects the blood vessels and internal organs. This condition is characterized by various symptoms, including fragile blood vessels, thin and translucent skin, easy bruising, and joint hypermobility. Most significantly, individuals with vEDS face an increased risk of life-threatening complications, such as arterial or organ rupture, highlighting the importance of early diagnosis and management.

Unlocking the Genetic Code:
The Science Behind vEDS

Like other forms of EDS, vEDS is an inherited condition passed down through families. It is an autosomal dominant disorder, meaning that an individual only needs to inherit one copy of the mutated gene from one parent to develop the condition. The gene responsible for vEDS is called COL3A1, which encodes the pro-alpha1(III) chain of type III collagen. Mutations in the COL3A1 gene result in the production of structurally abnormal collagen, leading to the various symptoms associated with vEDS.

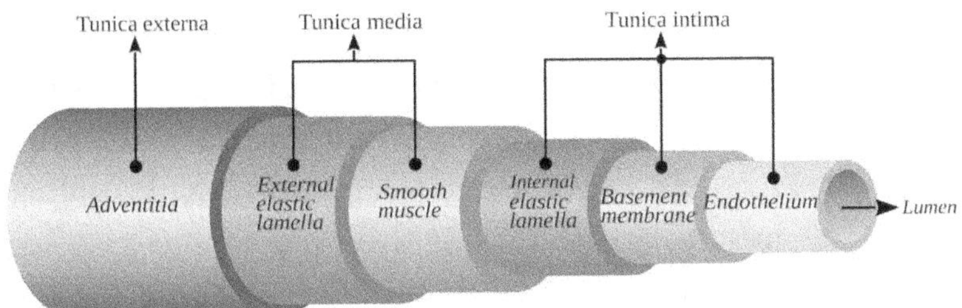

In general, the blood vessel wall has three layers, which are named from outside to inside how: tunica externa, tunica media and tunica intima.

HYPERMOBILE EDS

Hypermobile EDS (hEDS) is a genetic disorder that affects the body's connective tissues, which provide support to the skin, bones, blood vessels, and other organs. People with hEDS often have loose, unstable joints, making them more prone to dislocations and chronic pain. The condition can also impact the skin, causing it to be more elastic and prone to bruising. While hEDS primarily affects the joints and skin, it can also involve other body systems, leading to a wide range of symptoms and challenges.

Symptoms and Challenges of hEDS

Individuals with hEDS can experience a variety of symptoms, some of which may include:

1. **Joint hypermobility:** A hallmark feature of hEDS, joint hypermobility is characterized by an unusually large range of motion in the affected joints. This can lead to joint instability, frequent dislocations, and chronic pain.
2. **Soft, hyper-elastic skin:** Many people with hEDS have skin that is soft to the touch and can stretch more than usual. This increased elasticity can make the skin more prone to injury and bruising.
3. **Chronic pain:** Due to joint instability and frequent dislocations, individuals with hEDS often experience chronic pain, which can impact their daily life and mental well-being.
4. **Fatigue:** Chronic pain and other symptoms of hEDS can contribute to persistent fatigue, making it difficult for those with the condition to maintain a normal level of activity.
5. **Gastrointestinal issues:** Some individuals with hEDS may also experience gastrointestinal symptoms, such as acid reflux, constipation, and irritable bowel syndrome (IBS).

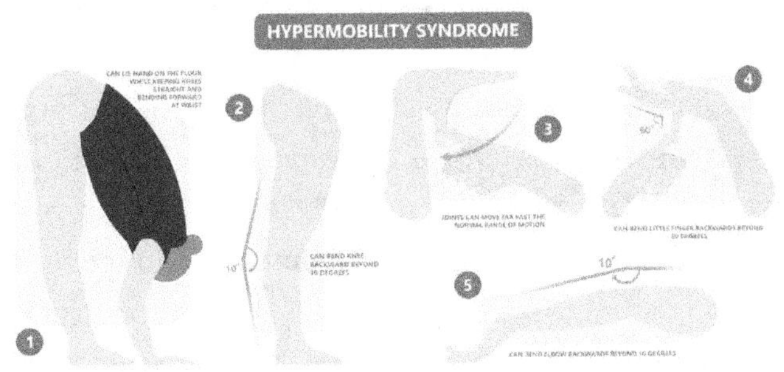

ARTHROCHALASIA EDS

Arthrochalasia EDS (aEDS) is a subtype of EDS, characterized by severe joint hypermobility, frequent dislocations, and congenital hip dislocation. The word "arthrochalasia" itself is derived from the Greek words for "joint" and "relaxation," which aptly describes the main symptoms of this condition. Individuals with aEDS often experience recurrent joint dislocations, muscle weakness, and joint pain.

Root Causes and Diagnosis

Arthrochalasia EDS is caused by genetic mutations that affect the production of collagen, a critical protein in the body's connective tissues. Specifically, these mutations occur in the genes known as COL1A1 and COL1A2, which encode for type I collagen. Collagen provides strength and elasticity to various tissues, including skin, ligaments, and tendons.

Diagnosing aEDS can be challenging due to its rarity and overlapping clinical features with other types of EDS. Genetic testing is typically utilized to confirm the diagnosis. Comprehensive clinical assessments, including physical examinations and detailed patient history, are also crucial in determining the appropriate course of action for patients.

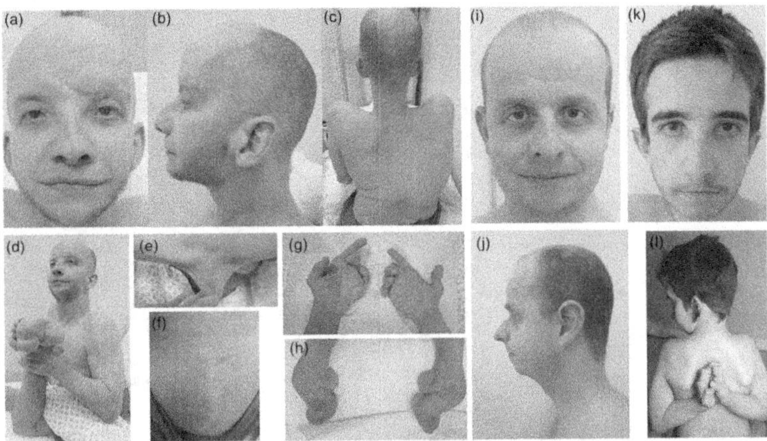

Clinical features of patients with aEDS. a–h (P1). (a) Hypertelorism, blue sclerae, scar on forehead after a fall. (b) Depressed nasal bridge. (c) Scoliosis. (d) Increased endorotation of the left hip joint and deformed foot with wrinkling of the sole. (e) Skin hyperextensibility. (f) Wide scar. (g) Hypermobile phalangeal joints with flexion contractures of multiple fingers and wrinkling of the palms. (h) Severe cavus deformation of both feet. i,j (P3). White sclerae, absence of hypertelorism. (j) Depressed nasal bridge and micrognathia. k,l (P5). Blue sclerae and micrognathia (l) Generalized joint hypermobility, hearing aid, scar from spinal surgery (Ayoub, S et al. Am J Med Genet Part A. 2020).

DERMATOSPARAXIS EDS

Dermatosparaxis EDS (dEDS) is a rare subtype of a group of genetic disorders that affect the connective tissues in the body. The term "dermatosparaxis" is derived from the Greek words for "skin" and "tear," which aptly describe one of the key symptoms of this condition. Individuals with dEDS often experience fragile skin that is prone to tearing, bruising, and scarring.

<h2 style="text-align:center">Symptoms and Clinical Features</h2>

The primary symptoms of dEDS include:

- Extremely fragile skin that tears and bruises easily
- Sagging, redundant skin, often described as "doughy" or "velvety" to the touch
- Delayed wound healing and abnormal scarring
- Joint hypermobility, particularly in small joints like fingers and toes
- Hernias and organ prolapse

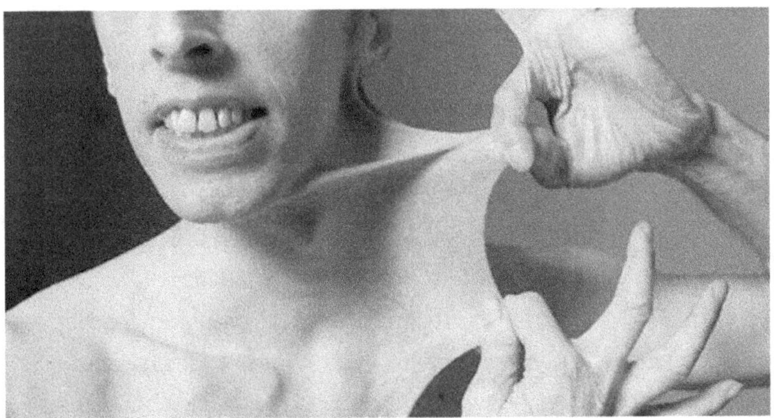

The severity of symptoms can vary significantly among individuals. However, the hallmark features of fragile skin and joint hypermobility are typically present to some degree in all cases.

KYPHOSCOLIOTIC EDS

Our body's connective tissue is a vital component that provides support, structure, and strength to various organs, bones, and muscles. Kyphoscoliotic EDS (kEDS) is caused by mutations in the PLOD1 or FKBP14 genes, leading to a deficiency in the enzyme lysyl hydroxylase 1 (LH1) or a defect in the protein FKBP14. This results in abnormal collagen formation, causing the connective tissue to become weak and fragile.

The term "kyphoscoliotic" refers to two characteristic features of this subtype: kyphosis (an exaggerated forward rounding of the upper back) and scoliosis (a sideways curvature of the spine). However, kEDS affects not only the spine but also a wide range of other bodily systems.

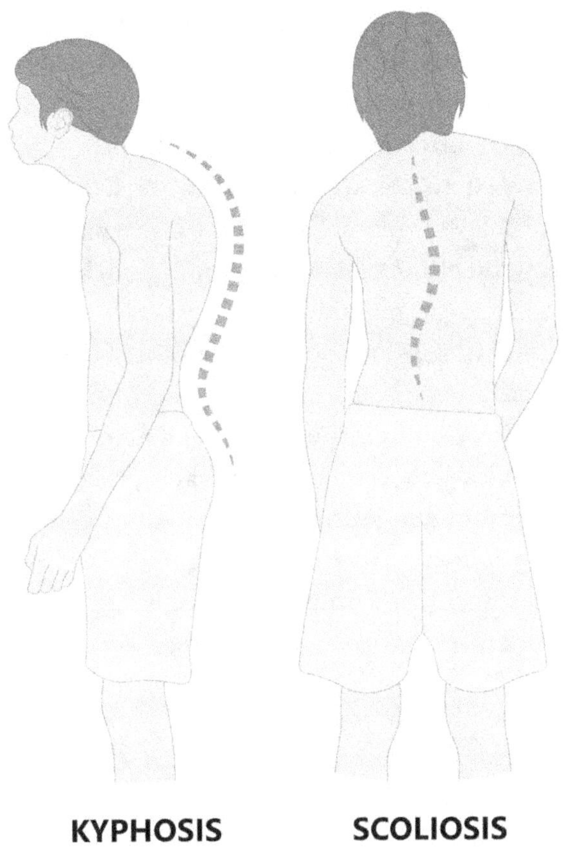

Spine curvature disorders

Symptoms and Complications

Kyphoscoliotic EDS affects individuals differently, but common symptoms and complications include:

- **Joint hypermobility:** The increased flexibility of joints can lead to frequent dislocations, sprains, and pain.

- **Muscle hypotonia:** Decreased muscle tone may cause delayed motor development, fatigue, and muscle weakness.
- **Skin manifestations:** The skin may be hyperextensible, soft, and easily bruised. Scarring and delayed wound healing are also common.
- **Skeletal abnormalities:** In addition to kyphosis and scoliosis, individuals may experience early-onset arthritis, osteoporosis, or other bone deformities.
- **Cardiovascular issues:** Heart and blood vessel complications, such as mitral valve prolapse or aortic root dilation, may occur.
- **Eye problems:** Myopia (nearsightedness), retinal detachment, and other vision issues are possible.

SPONDYLO-DYSPLASTIC EDS

Spondylodysplastic EDS (spEDS) is a rare subtype of EDS, characterized by short stature, muscle hypotonia, and skeletal dysplasia. This condition affects the connective tissues, which play a crucial role in providing support and structure to various parts of the body, such as the skin, blood vessels, and bones.

Individuals with spEDS often experience a range of symptoms that can vary in severity, including joint hypermobility, skin hyperextensibility, and delayed motor development. In addition, this condition can lead to a number of complications, such as scoliosis, joint dislocations, and chronic pain.

The Genetic Basis of spEDS

Spondylodysplastic EDS is caused by genetic mutations that affect the production of certain proteins involved in the formation and maintenance of connective tissues. Specifically, these mutations occur in the genes B4GALT7, B3GALT6, and SLC39A13, which are responsible for the synthesis of important components of the extracellular matrix, such as proteoglycans and glycosaminoglycans.

This condition is inherited in an autosomal recessive manner, meaning that an individual must inherit two copies of the mutated gene (one from each parent) to be affected. Parents who are carriers of the mutation have a 25% chance of having a child with spEDS.

MUSCULO-CONTRACTURAL EDS

Musculocontractural EDS (mcEDS) is a rare subtype of EDS characterized by congenital multiple contractures, distinctive craniofacial features, and progressive joint and skin involvement. This condition affects the connective tissues, which are responsible for providing support and structure to various parts of the body, such as the skin, blood vessels, and bones.

Individuals with mcEDS often experience a range of symptoms, including joint hypermobility, skin hyperextensibility, and muscle hypotonia. In addition, they may have unique craniofacial features, such as a prominent forehead, down-slanting palpebral fissures, and a small mouth.

MYOPATHIC EDS

Myopathic EDS (mEDS) is a rare subtype of EDS, characterized by congenital muscle hypotonia, muscle atrophy, and joint hypermobility. This condition affects the connective tissues that provide support and structure to various parts of the body, such as the skin, blood vessels, and bones.

Individuals with mEDS often experience a range of symptoms, including muscle weakness, joint instability, and delayed motor development. In some cases, affected individuals may also have mild hyperextensibility of the skin.

The Genetic Basis of mEDS

Myopathic EDS is caused by genetic mutations that affect the production of certain proteins involved in the formation and maintenance of connective tissues. Specifically, these mutations occur in the genes COL12A1 and FKBP14, which are responsible for encoding proteins essential for the proper functioning of the extracellular matrix.

This condition is inherited in an autosomal recessive manner, meaning that an individual must inherit two copies of the mutated gene (one from each parent) to be affected. Parents who are carriers of the mutation have a 25% chance of having a child with Myopathic EDS.

PERIODONTAL EDS

Periodontal EDS (pEDS) is a rare subtype of EDS, characterized by severe periodontal inflammation, early tooth loss, and connective tissue abnormalities. This condition affects the connective tissues that provide support and structure to various parts of the body, such as the skin, blood vessels, and bones.

Individuals with pEDS often experience a range of symptoms, including severe gum inflammation, premature loss of primary and permanent teeth, and an increased risk of oral infections. In some cases, affected individuals may also exhibit skin manifestations, such as easy bruising and slow wound healing.

The Genetic Basis of pEDS

Periodontal EDS is caused by genetic mutations that affect the production of certain proteins involved in the formation and maintenance of connective tissues. Specifically, these mutations occur in the C1R and C1S genes, which are responsible for encoding proteins essential for the proper functioning of the complement system, a crucial component of the immune system.

This condition is inherited in an autosomal dominant manner, meaning that an individual only needs to inherit one copy of the mutated gene from one parent to be affected. Parents with the mutation have a 50% chance of passing it on to their child.

SYMPTOMS AND CLINICAL FEATURES

COMMON SIGNS AND SYMPTOMS

While each subtype of EDS has its own unique set of symptoms and clinical features, there are some common signs and symptoms that are shared across the different subtypes. These include:

JOINT HYPERMOBILITY

Joint hypermobility is a hallmark feature of EDS and refers to an increased range of motion in the joints. This can lead to joint pain, instability, and a higher risk of dislocations and subluxations (partial dislocations).

SKIN MANIFESTATIONS

Individuals with EDS often have skin that is hyper-elastic, meaning it can be stretched more than normal. The skin may also be fragile and prone to bruising and scarring easily.

CARDIOVASCULAR COMPLICATIONS

Some forms of EDS can cause cardiovascular complications, such as heart valve abnormalities, aortic dilation, and an increased risk of arterial rupture.

MUSCULOSKELETAL ISSUES

Muscle weakness and pain, as well as early-onset osteoarthritis, can be common in individuals with EDS.

GASTROINTESTINAL SYMPTOMS

Gastrointestinal issues, including functional gastrointestinal disorders like irritable bowel syndrome (IBS), are commonly reported in people with EDS.

NEUROLOGICAL COMPLICATIONS

Neurological issues, such as headaches, migraines, and neuropathic pain, can also be present in individuals with EDS.

SUBTYPE-SPECIFIC SYMPTOMS AND CLINICAL FEATURES

In this section, we will delve into the specific symptoms and clinical features of each EDS subtype. This will provide a more detailed understanding of the unique characteristics of each subtype.

CLASSICAL EDS (CEDS)

Classical EDS is characterized by:

- Joint hypermobility, particularly in the fingers, wrists, and elbows
- Highly elastic, fragile, and easily bruised skin
- Atrophic (thin) scarring, especially over pressure points
- Soft, doughy skin texture
- Molluscoid pseudotumors (fleshy, noncancerous growths) and subcutaneous spheroids (hard, spherical nodules under the skin)

CLASSICAL-LIKE EDS (CLEDS)

Classical-like EDS (clEDS) is similar to cEDS but has some distinct differences:

- Joint hypermobility, though generally less severe than in cEDS
- Elastic skin, but with less pronounced scarring
- Skin that is more prone to bruising
- Absence of atrophic scarring

CARDIAC-VALVULAR EDS (CVEDS)

Cardiac-valvular EDS (cvEDS) primarily affects the heart and blood vessels and is characterized by:

- Severe, progressive heart valve problems, particularly affecting the mitral and aortic valves
- Joint hypermobility, but typically limited to the small joints of the hands
- Skin that may be slightly more elastic and fragile than normal

VASCULAR EDS (VEDS)

Vascular EDS (vEDS) is the most serious form of EDS due to its life-threatening complications. It is characterized by:

- Thin, translucent skin with visible veins, particularly on the chest and abdomen
- Fragile blood vessels and a high risk of arterial rupture, leading to life-threatening internal bleeding

- An increased risk of organ rupture, such as the intestines or uterus during pregnancy
- Joint hypermobility, typically limited to the small joints of the hands and feet

HYPERMOBILE EDS (HEDS)

Hypermobile EDS (hEDS) is the most common subtype of EDS and is characterized by:

- Generalized joint hypermobility, affecting both large and small joints
- Chronic joint pain and a higher risk of dislocations and subluxations
- Soft, smooth skin that may be slightly more elastic than normal
- Gastrointestinal issues, such as IBS, and autonomic dysfunction, which affects the regulation of heart rate, blood pressure, and digestion

ARTHROCHALASIA EDS (AEDS)

Arthrochalasia EDS (aEDS) is a rare subtype characterized by:

- Severe joint hypermobility, leading to frequent dislocations and subluxations, particularly of the hips
- Congenital hip dislocation (present at birth)
- Elastic, fragile skin with a tendency to bruise easily
- Atrophic scarring and delayed wound healing

DERMATOSPARAXIS EDS (DEDS)

Dermatosparaxis EDS (dEDS) is a rare subtype characterized by:

- Extremely fragile skin that is prone to tearing and bruising easily
- Redundant, sagging skin, particularly on the face
- Joint hypermobility, particularly in the hands
- Delayed closure of the fontanelles (soft spots on a baby's skull)

KYPHOSCOLIOTIC EDS (KEDS)

Kyphoscoliotic EDS (kEDS) is characterized by:

- Progressive kyphoscoliosis (an abnormal curvature of the spine in both the sagittal and coronal planes)
- Severe muscle hypotonia (low muscle tone) at birth, which may improve with age
- Joint hypermobility, particularly in the hands and feet
- Fragile, elastic skin with a tendency to bruise easily

SPONDYLODYSPLASTIC EDS (SPEDS)

Spondylodysplastic EDS (spEDS) is characterized by:

- Short stature and skeletal abnormalities, such as abnormal curvature of the spine and malformed bones
- Joint hypermobility, particularly in the hands and feet
- Soft, doughy skin with a tendency to bruise easily
- Mild to moderate intellectual disability or learning difficulties

MUSCULOCONTRACTURAL EDS (MCEDS)

Musculocontractural EDS (mcEDS) is characterized by:

- Congenital multiple contractures (joints that are fixed in a bent or straightened position)
- Joint hypermobility
- Characteristic facial features, such as a small chin, large eyes, and a thin upper lip
- Skin that is prone to bruising and scarring

MYOPATHIC EDS (MEDS)

Myopathic EDS (mEDS) is characterized by:

- Muscle weakness and hypotonia, particularly affecting the proximal muscles (those closest to the body's center)
- Joint hypermobility, particularly in the hands and feet

- Skin that may be slightly more elastic and fragile
  than normal

PERIODONTAL EDS (PEDS)

Periodontal EDS (pEDS) is characterized by:

- Severe gum disease (periodontitis), leading to early
  tooth loss
- Joint hypermobility, particularly in the hands
- Skin that may be slightly more elastic and fragile
  than normal

DIAGNOSIS OF EHLERS-DANLOS SYNDROME

EDS is a complex group of heritable connective tissue disorders, comprising 13 subtypes with varying clinical presentations. Diagnosing EDS can be challenging due to the wide range of symptoms and the overlap with other conditions. In this chapter, we will discuss the available methods and tools for diagnosing EDS, such as clinical assessment, genetic testing, and diagnostic criteria. We will also explore the value of each method in terms of their potential for false positives or negatives, providing a comprehensive analysis that caters to a general audience.

CLINICAL ASSESSMENT

Clinical assessment is the first step in diagnosing EDS and involves a thorough evaluation of the patient's medical history, physical examination, and, in some cases, specialist consultations. This section will discuss the various aspects of clinical assessment and their significance in the diagnosis of EDS.

MEDICAL HISTORY

A comprehensive medical history is vital in the diagnostic process of EDS. It involves gathering information about the patient's symptoms, their onset and progression, family history of EDS or related connective tissue disorders, and any previous surgeries or medical interventions. This information helps clinicians identify patterns and features suggestive of EDS and guides further evaluation.

PHYSICAL EXAMINATION

A thorough physical examination is crucial for identifying signs and symptoms consistent with EDS. Key areas of focus include:

- **Joint mobility:** Assessing joint hypermobility using tests such as the Beighton Score or the Five-Point Questionnaire for Hypermobility.
- **Skin examination:** Evaluating the skin for hyperextensibility, fragility, unusual scarring, and bruising.
- **Musculoskeletal assessment:** Looking for muscle weakness, pain, or early-onset osteoarthritis.
- **Cardiovascular examination:** Checking for heart murmurs, which may indicate valvular abnormalities, and assessing blood pressure and heart rate for signs of autonomic dysfunction.

SPECIALIST CONSULTATIONS

In some cases, specialist consultations may be necessary to further evaluate specific symptoms or to rule out other conditions with similar clinical presentations. For example, a cardiologist may assess potential cardiovascular complications, while a geneticist may provide guidance on genetic testing.

GENETIC TESTING

Genetic testing is an essential tool in the diagnosis of most EDS subtypes, as it can identify pathogenic variants in specific genes associated with the condition. This section will discuss the various genetic testing methods and their role in diagnosing EDS.

TARGETED GENE TESTING

Targeted gene testing involves analyzing specific genes known to be associated with EDS subtypes. This method is particularly useful when a clinical assessment strongly suggests a particular EDS subtype, and the corresponding gene can be tested for pathogenic variants. However, this approach may not be as helpful when the clinical presentation is ambiguous, or multiple genes may be involved.

PANEL TESTING

Panel testing involves analyzing multiple genes simultaneously, which can be beneficial in cases where the clinical presentation is not specific to a single EDS subtype. By testing for several genes associated with EDS and related connective tissue disorders, panel testing can increase the likelihood of identifying the underlying genetic cause. However, this method may also identify variants of uncertain significance (VUS) that require further evaluation to determine their relevance to the patient's symptoms.

WHOLE EXOME OR WHOLE GENOME SEQUENCING

Whole exome or whole genome sequencing involves analyzing the entire protein-coding region (exome) or the entire DNA sequence (genome) of an individual. While these methods can potentially identify novel genetic causes of EDS, their use is generally limited to research settings or cases where targeted gene testing and panel testing have not provided a diagnosis.

Genetic Sequencing: Pros and Cons

	Whole Exome and Whole Genome Sequencing	Gene Panel	Targeted Single Gene
PROS	• More comprehensive test • Can reduce diagnostic odyssey • Possible to reanalyze data later	• Shorter turnaround time than exome • Lower cost than exome • Can sequence many genes at once	• Quicker turnaround time • Lower cost • Easy analysis • No secondary or incidental findings
CONS	• Longer turnaround time • Higher cost • Secondary and incidental findings possible • Higher chance of uncertain result	• Can miss diagnosis if gene isn't on the panel • Reanalysis not possible • Higher cost than targeted test	• Must know gene of interest • Lower ability to detect novel variants

DIAGNOSTIC CRITERIA

Diagnostic criteria are essential for standardizing the diagnosis of EDS and ensuring that clinicians and researchers are consistent in their identification of the condition. The 2017 International Classification of EDS outlines the diagnostic criteria for each EDS subtype, incorporating clinical features, family history, and genetic testing results. This section will discuss the various components of the diagnostic criteria and their significance in accurately diagnosing EDS.

MAJOR AND MINOR CRITERIA

The diagnostic criteria for each EDS subtype include major and minor criteria. Major criteria are clinical features with a high specificity for a particular subtype, while minor criteria are less specific but may support the diagnosis when present. A combination of major and minor criteria is typically necessary to establish a diagnosis.

FAMILY HISTORY

Family history is an important component of the diagnostic criteria, as EDS is an inherited condition. In some cases, a positive family history of EDS or related connective tissue disorders can support the diagnosis, particularly when the clinical presentation is less clear-cut.

GENETIC TESTING

Genetic testing results are incorporated into the diagnostic criteria for most EDS subtypes. The identification of a pathogenic variant in a gene associated with a specific EDS subtype can confirm the diagnosis. However, it is essential to consider the clinical context when interpreting genetic testing results to avoid false positives or negatives.

FALSE POSITIVES AND FALSE NEGATIVES

Accurate diagnosis of EDS is critical for appropriate management and treatment. However, the potential for false positives and false negatives exists in each diagnostic method. This section will discuss the factors contributing to false positives and false negatives and their implications for the diagnosis of EDS.

CLINICAL ASSESSMENT

False positives in clinical assessment can occur when symptoms mimic those of EDS, leading to overdiagnosis. For example, joint hypermobility may be present in other connective tissue disorders or as a normal variant in some individuals. Similarly, skin hyperextensibility and easy bruising can be observed in other conditions or as a result of certain medications. To minimize false positives, it is essential to consider the entire clinical presentation and to rule out alternative diagnoses.

False negatives in clinical assessment can occur when

symptoms are mild or atypical, leading to underdiagnosis. This can be particularly challenging in EDS subtypes with less specific clinical features or those that present later in life. To minimize false negatives, a thorough and comprehensive assessment is necessary, and referral to specialists may be needed for further evaluation.

GENETIC TESTING

False positives in genetic testing can occur when a variant of uncertain significance (VUS) is misinterpreted as pathogenic, leading to overdiagnosis. To minimize false positives, it is essential to consider the clinical context and to seek expert guidance in interpreting genetic testing results.

False negatives in genetic testing can occur when the pathogenic variant is not identified due to limitations in the testing method or when the underlying genetic cause of EDS is not yet known. To minimize false negatives, it is important to consider the entire clinical presentation and to pursue further testing or specialist consultations when indicated.

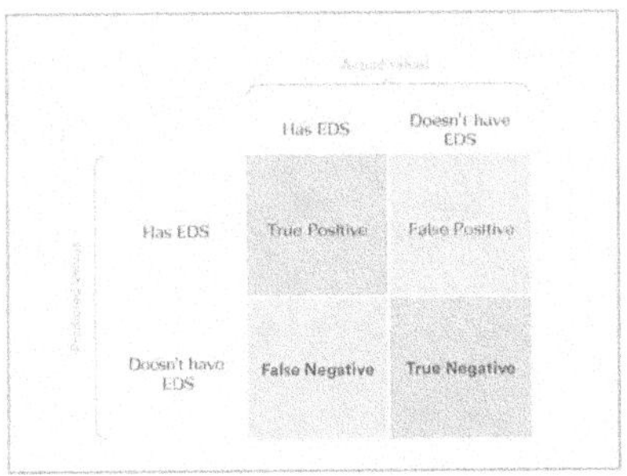

MANAGEMENT AND TREATMENT

Management and treatment of EDS requires a multidisciplinary approach, combining physical therapy, pain management, surgical interventions, and psychological support. By tailoring treatment strategies to the specific needs of each individual, healthcare professionals can help improve the quality of life for people living with EDS and their families. While living with EDS can be challenging, with appropriate management and support, affected individuals can lead fulfilling lives.

PHYSICAL THERAPY

ROLE OF PHYSICAL THERAPY IN EDS MANAGEMENT

Physical therapy is a crucial component of EDS management. It focuses on improving joint stability, muscle strength, and proprioception, which is the body's ability to sense its position in space. Physical therapy can also help to prevent injuries and manage pain.

TYPES OF PHYSICAL THERAPY TECHNIQUES

Strengthening Exercises: These exercises aim to increase muscle strength around the joints, providing additional support and reducing joint instability. Examples include resistance training with bands or weights and isometric exercises.

Range of Motion Exercises: These exercises help maintain joint flexibility and prevent stiffness. Examples include gentle stretching and joint mobilization techniques.

Proprioceptive Training: This type of training is designed to improve body awareness and coordination. Examples include balance exercises, coordination drills, and activities using stability balls or wobble boards.

Aquatic Therapy: Aquatic therapy involves performing exercises in a pool, which provides buoyancy and reduces the impact on joints. This can be beneficial for EDS patients with significant joint pain or instability.

CONSIDERATIONS FOR PHYSICAL THERAPY IN EDS PATIENTS

When designing a physical therapy program for individuals with EDS, therapists must be aware of the specific needs and limitations of EDS patients. Overstretching should be avoided, as it can further damage the already fragile connective tissues. Additionally, progress should be gradual to prevent injury and allow for sufficient recovery time.

PAIN MANAGEMENT

Pain in EDS can be multifaceted, often resulting from joint dislocations, muscle spasms, nerve pain, and inflammation. Pain can vary in intensity and duration, and it can significantly impact a person's quality of life, often leading to reduced mobility and function. Given the complexity and chronic nature of pain in EDS, effective pain management is essential.

CONVENTIONAL AND NON-CONVENTIONAL PAIN MANAGEMENT STRATEGIES

Pain management in EDS often involves a multidisciplinary approach, incorporating both pharmacological and non-pharmacological strategies.

Pharmacological treatments can include over-the-counter analgesics like NSAIDs, acetaminophen, or prescribed medications like opioids, depending on the severity of the pain. However, these need to be used judiciously due to potential side effects and the risk of dependency, particularly with long-term use.

Non-pharmacological interventions can be equally, if not more, important. These may involve physical therapy to strengthen muscles and stabilize joints, occupational therapy to help modify activities and environments, and psychological therapies like cognitive-behavioral therapy to help manage the emotional impact of chronic pain.

Additionally, some patients may find benefit from complementary therapies such as acupuncture, massage, or hydrotherapy.

THE IMPORTANCE OF PERSONALIZED TREATMENT PLANS

Given the wide variability in the presentation and severity of EDS, there is no one-size-fits-all approach to pain management. A personalized treatment plan, developed in collaboration with a healthcare provider, can help ensure that pain management strategies are tailored to the individual's needs and circumstances. Regular review and adjustment of this plan are crucial to ensure its continued effectiveness and to address any new or worsening symptoms.

SURGICAL INTERVENTIONS

Surgical intervention for patients with EDS is often considered a last resort due to the potential complications associated with the disease and surgical procedures. The primary objective is to alleviate pain, prevent or manage complications, and improve the patient's quality of life. Here's a more detailed look at the role of surgery in the treatment of EDS:

PAIN MANAGEMENT

Significant, chronic pain is a common symptom in individuals with EDS. When conservative pain management methods such as medication, physical therapy, and lifestyle modifications do not provide sufficient relief, surgery may be considered. For instance, orthopedic surgeries like joint replacements or fusions can help alleviate joint pain and improve stability.

PREVENTING AND MANAGING COMPLICATIONS

EDS can lead to various complications such as joint disloca-tions, spine instability, heart problems, or digestive system issues. In some cases, these complications may necessitate surgical intervention. For instance, cardiovascular surgery may be required to repair or replace a damaged heart valve in cases of vascular EDS.

IMPROVING FUNCTION AND STABILITY

In some patients, the joint instability associated with EDS can lead to difficulty in performing daily activities and maintaining independence. Surgical interventions can improve joint stability and, consequently, enhance the patient's function and independence.

LIMITATIONS AND RISKS

Surgery in EDS patients is not without risks. The disorder's hallmark traits—elastic skin and overly flexible joints—can complicate both the procedure and the healing process. Surgeons must handle tissues gently and suture meticulously to avoid causing damage. Healing may be slower and scar formation may be unusual due to the nature of the connective tissue in EDS.

Given these risks, comprehensive pre-surgical evaluations are important. The decision to proceed with surgery should be made after careful consideration and discussion between the patient and a multidisciplinary team of healthcare providers, including surgeons knowledgeable about EDS.

JOINT SURGERY

Joint instability and associated pain are common problems in people with EDS. When conservative treatment options like physical therapy, braces, or pain management do not provide sufficient relief, joint surgery may be considered. However, it's important to note that due to the nature of EDS, surgery should be approached with caution and patients should be managed by a team familiar with the condition.

INDICATIONS FOR JOINT SURGERY

The primary indications for joint surgery in patients with EDS include:

- **Chronic Pain:** Intractable, chronic pain that significantly impairs quality of life and does not respond to non-surgical treatments may indicate the need for joint surgery.

- **Joint Instability:** Frequent dislocations or subluxations that lead to functional impairment might necessitate surgical intervention.
- **Joint Damage:** Significant joint damage seen on imaging studies, often the result of repeated dislocations or wear-and-tear, can indicate the need for surgery.

PROCEDURES

The specific surgical procedure will depend on the joint involved and the patient's specific symptoms and overall health status. Some common joint surgeries include:

Arthroscopy: This is a minimally invasive procedure used to diagnose and treat problems in a joint. The surgeon inserts a small camera, called an arthroscope, into the joint through a small incision. The camera displays pictures on a television screen, and the surgeon uses these images to guide miniature surgical instruments.

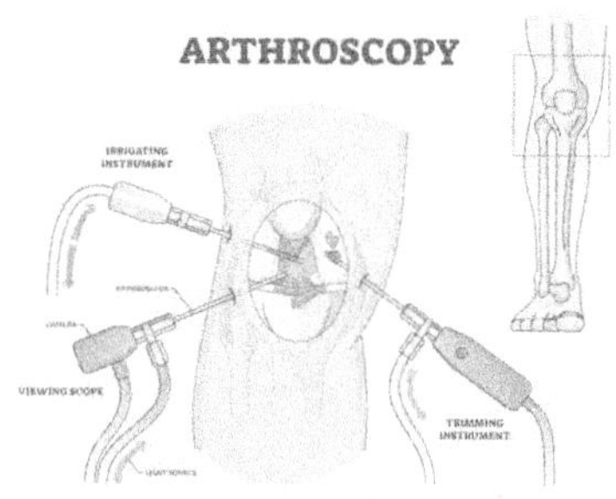

Arthroplasty: Also known as joint replacement, this procedure involves removing a damaged joint and replacing it with an artificial one. Hip and knee replacements are the most commonly performed joint replacements, but this procedure can also be performed on other joints, like the shoulder, elbow, wrist, or ankle.

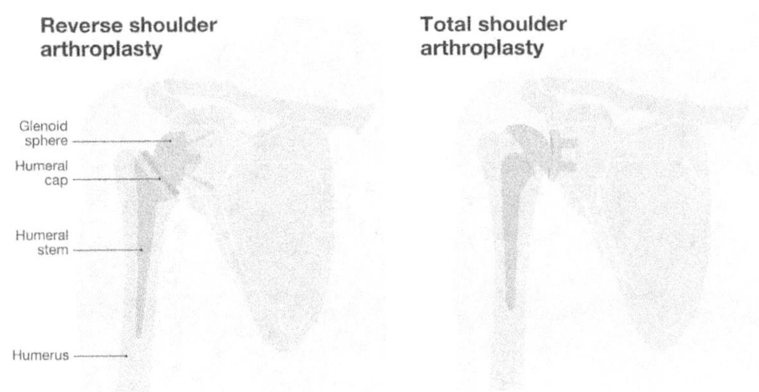

Arthrodesis: Also known as joint fusion, this procedure involves merging the bones of the joint together. This can improve stability and reduce pain but at the expense of joint mobility. This procedure is commonly performed on the spine but can also be done on other joints like the wrist or ankle.

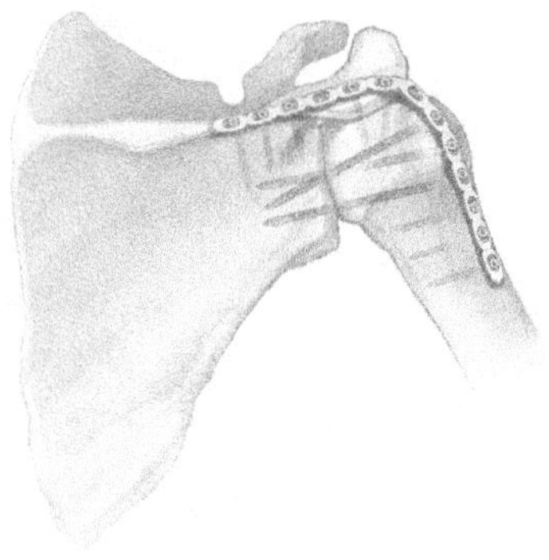

Tendon Repair or Transfer: These procedures can help improve joint stability and function. Tendon repair involves using sutures to bring a torn tendon back together, while tendon transfer involves moving a tendon from its original attachment to a new one to restore function.

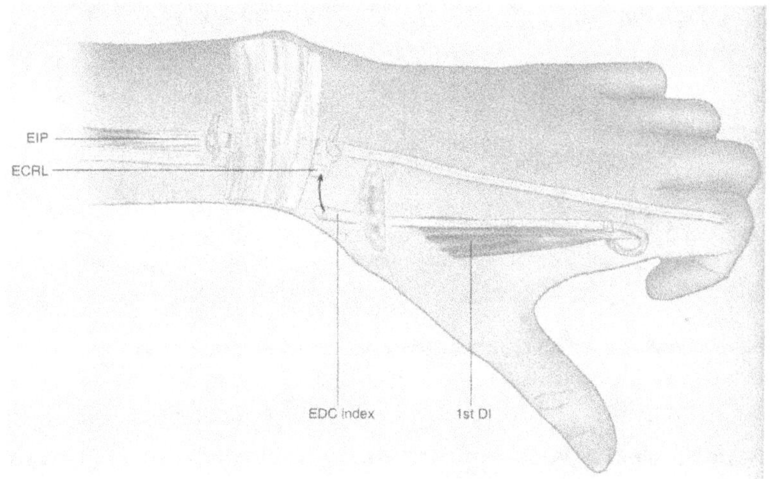

Each of these procedures has its own risks and benefits, and the choice of procedure will depend on a variety of factors such as the severity of the joint damage, the patient's age and overall health, and the surgeon's expertise. The surgeon and patient should discuss these factors thoroughly before making a decision.

SPINAL SURGERY

EDS can affect the spine, leading to conditions like scoliosis (abnormal curvature of the spine), kyphosis (forward bending of the spine), and craniocervical instability (instability of the junction of the skull and neck). In some cases, these conditions may necessitate surgical intervention. However, due to the complexity of EDS and the potential risks associated with surgery, these procedures should be performed by a surgical team experienced in treating patients with EDS.

INDICATIONS FOR SPINAL SURGERY

The primary indications for spinal surgery in patients with EDS include:

1. **Pain:** Chronic, severe back pain that does not respond to conservative treatments may indicate the need for spinal surgery.
2. **Neurological Impairment:** Conditions like craniocervical instability can cause neurological symptoms, such as weakness, numbness, or impaired coordination. If these symptoms are severe or progressive, surgery may be necessary to prevent further neurologic damage.
3. **Progressive Deformity:** Progressive spinal deformities, such as worsening scoliosis or kyphosis, may require surgical correction to prevent further progression and associated complications.

PROCEDURES

The specific surgical procedure will depend on the part of the spine involved and the patient's specific symptoms and overall health status. Some common spinal surgeries include:

Spinal Fusion: This procedure is used to join two or more vertebrae together to improve stability, correct a deformity, or reduce pain. The surgeon uses bone grafts, and sometimes rods and screws, to encourage the vertebrae to grow together into one solid unit.

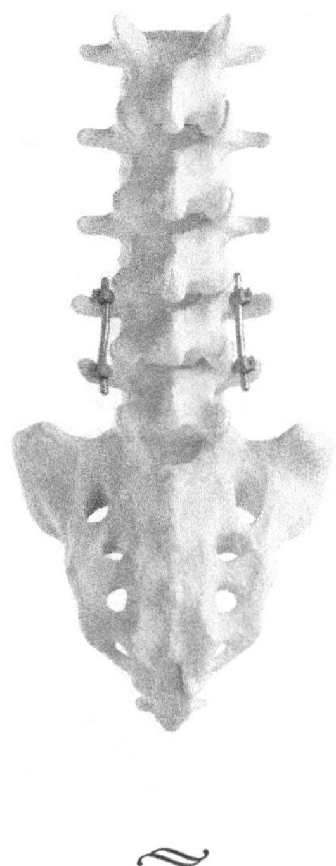

~

Decompression Surgery: This procedure involves removing structures that are pressing on the spinal cord or nerves, such as bone, disc material, or ligaments. This can relieve symptoms like pain, weakness, or numbness.

Lumbar Laminotomy and Discectomy

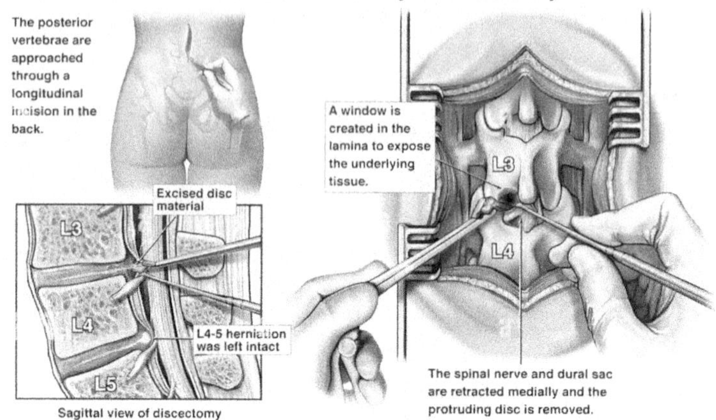

Sagittal view of discectomy

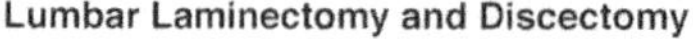

Lumbar Laminectomy and Discectomy

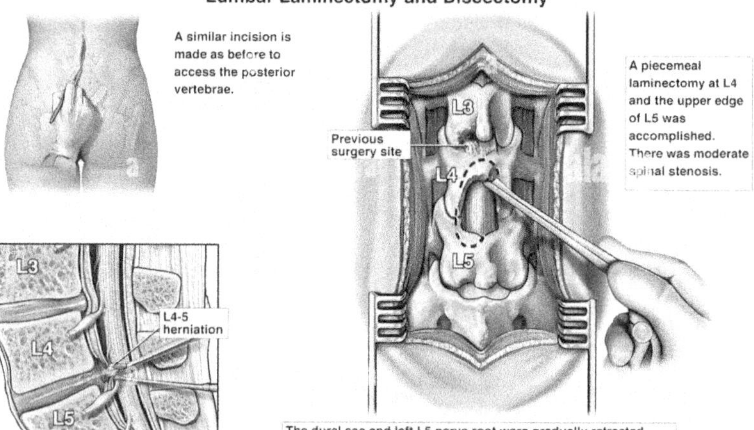

Sagittal view of discectomy

Craniocervical Fusion: In patients with craniocervical instability, a fusion of the skull and upper cervical spine can stabilize the area and prevent dangerous movement that could injure the spinal cord.

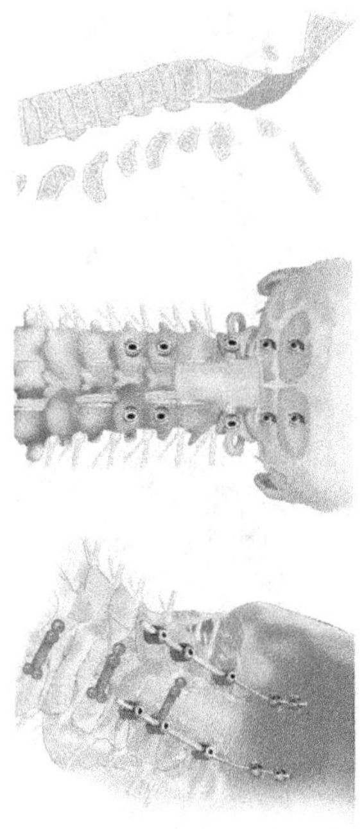

Scoliosis Surgery: For patients with significant scoliosis, a combination of spinal fusion and instrumentation (rods, screws) can be used to correct the curvature and stabilize the spine.

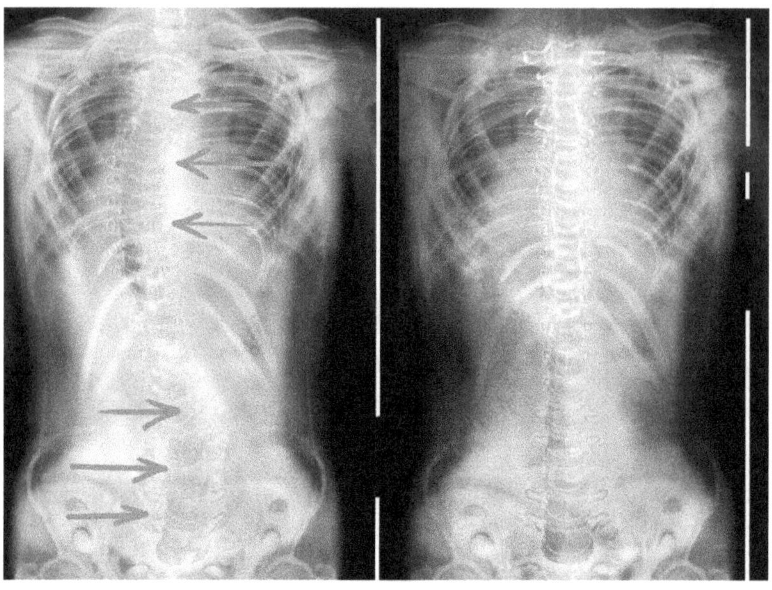

Each of these procedures has its own risks and benefits, and the choice of procedure will depend on a variety of factors. These include the severity of the spinal condition, the patient's age and overall health, and the surgeon's expertise. The surgeon and patient should discuss these factors thoroughly before making a decision.

REHABILITATION AFTER ORTHOPEDIC SURGERY!!!!!

After undergoing orthopedic surgery, patients with EDS will typically require a period of rehabilitation and physical therapy. This process is crucial for maximizing function, improving strength and flexibility, and enhancing overall recovery.

Rehabilitation and physical therapy can be broken down into several phases:

Immediate Postoperative Phase:

In the immediate postoperative phase, the focus is on pain management, wound care, and the prevention of complications such as blood clots. The patient may be instructed to perform gentle range-of-motion exercises to keep the joints flexible and promote circulation.

Early Rehabilitation:

As the patient heals, the focus of therapy will shift towards restoring function. This includes:

- **Range-of-Motion Exercises:** These exercises help maintain flexibility in the joints and prevent stiffness.

- **Strength Building:** Gradual strengthening exercises help rebuild muscles that may have weakened due to surgery or pre-surgical pain.
- **Gait Training:** For surgeries involving the lower extremities, like hip or knee surgeries, gait training can help patients regain the ability to walk correctly.

<u>Long-Term Rehabilitation:</u>

In the long-term phase, therapy will focus on further improving strength and flexibility, and on functional training to help the patient return to their daily activities. This can include:

- **Proprioceptive Training:** These exercises help improve the patient's awareness of their joint position, which can enhance stability and prevent further injury.
- **Functional and Occupational Therapy:** These therapies help patients relearn how to perform tasks necessary for daily life and work.
- **Pain Management:** Chronic pain can be a significant issue for patients with EDS. Therapists can provide strategies for managing pain, such as heat or ice therapy, massage, and relaxation techniques.

Throughout this process, the physical therapist will need to be aware of the patient's EDS diagnosis and adapt their approach accordingly. For example, because of the hypermobility associated with EDS, the therapist will need to ensure that exercises are safe and do not lead to joint injury.

Finally, it's important to note that the rehabilitation

process can be a long one, requiring significant commitment from the patient. The exact length and nature of the process will vary depending on the specific surgery performed, the patient's overall health, and the severity of their EDS symptoms.

Heart and Vascular Surgery

EDS, particularly the vascular type, can have significant implications for the cardiovascular system. The connective tissue abnormalities associated with EDS can lead to problems such as mitral valve prolapse, aortic root dilation, and in severe cases, arterial aneurysms and dissections. In some cases, these conditions may warrant surgical intervention.

INDICATIONS

Indications for heart and vascular surgery in patients with EDS include:

Cardiac Valve Dysfunction: Conditions such as mitral valve prolapse may progress to the point of causing significant valve leakage (regurgitation), which can lead to heart failure. In such cases, valve repair or replacement surgery may be necessary.

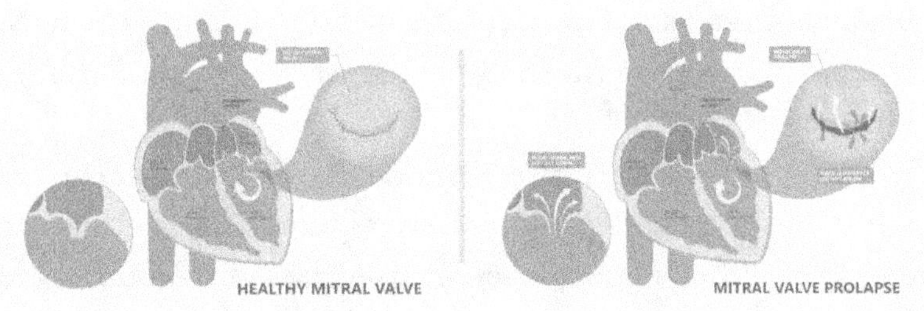

Aortic Root Dilation: Dilation of the aortic root can lead to aortic regurgitation or increase the risk of aortic dissection. If the aortic root becomes significantly dilated, surgical repair or replacement may be indicated.

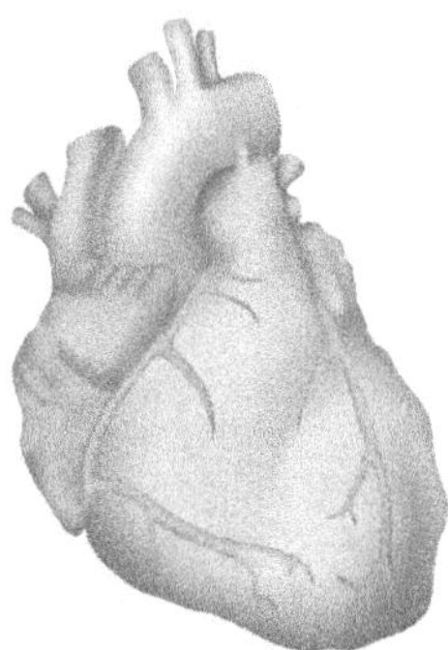

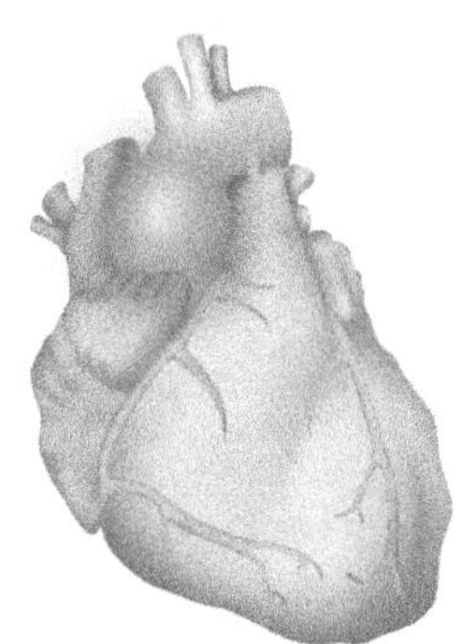

Arterial Aneurysms and Dissections: An arterial aneurysm is a bulging, weakened area in the wall of an artery. Over time, blood pressure can cause this weakened area to enlarge and potentially rupture, leading to life-threatening bleeding. Aneurysms can occur in any artery, but they're most common in the aorta (the body's main artery) and the arteries in the brain.

Aneurysms can be caused by a variety of factors, including high blood pressure, high cholesterol, smoking, and certain genetic conditions. Many aneurysms cause no symptoms and are only discovered during medical exams or imaging tests for other conditions. However, if an aneurysm ruptures, it can cause severe pain, a rapid heartbeat, and potentially deadly internal bleeding.

Arterial dissections occur when a tear forms in the inner

layer of an artery. When this happens, blood can get into the wall of the artery and separate (or dissect) the layers, causing the artery to bulge outward. This can decrease or even stop blood flow through the artery, or it can cause the artery to rupture.

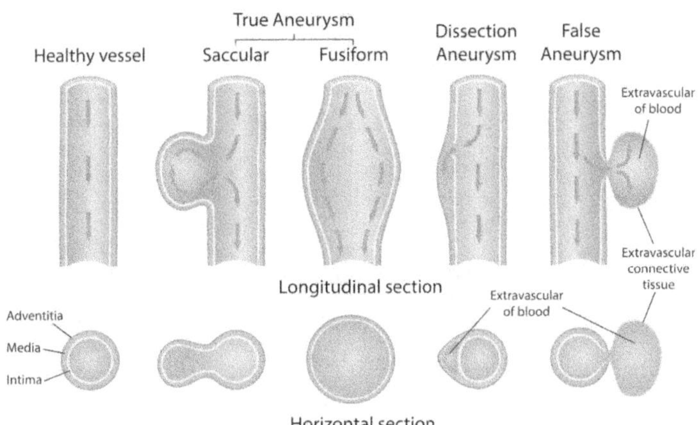

Arterial dissections can be caused by high blood pressure, injury to the artery, or certain genetic conditions. Symptoms can include severe pain, often described as a tearing or ripping sensation, that comes on suddenly. Depending on where the dissection occurs, other symptoms can include fainting, dizziness, stroke-like symptoms, or symptoms of a heart attack.

Both conditions are considered medical emergencies and require immediate treatment, which can include medication to lower blood pressure and prevent blood clots, or surgery to repair or replace the affected part of the artery.

PROCEDURES

The specific surgical procedure will depend on the cardiovascular problem at hand and the patient's overall health. Some common heart and vascular surgeries include:

Valve Repair or Replacement: Damaged or dysfunctional heart valves may need to be surgically repaired or replaced with a prosthetic valve.

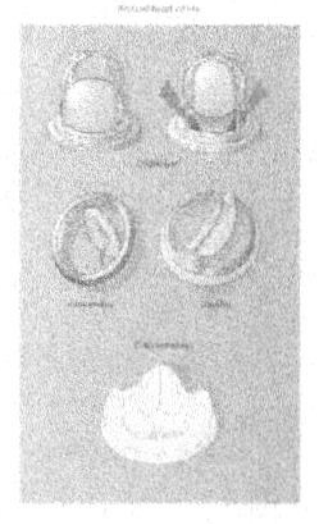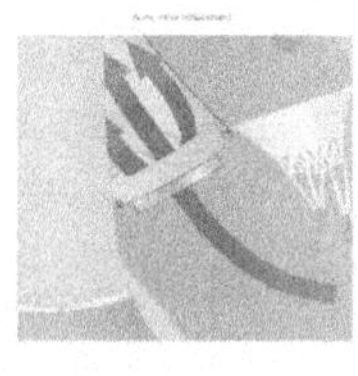

Aortic Root Repair or Replacement: If the aortic root is dilated or dissected, it may need to be repaired or replaced.

This is a complex procedure often involving the replacement of the aortic valve as well and is known as a "Bentall procedure".

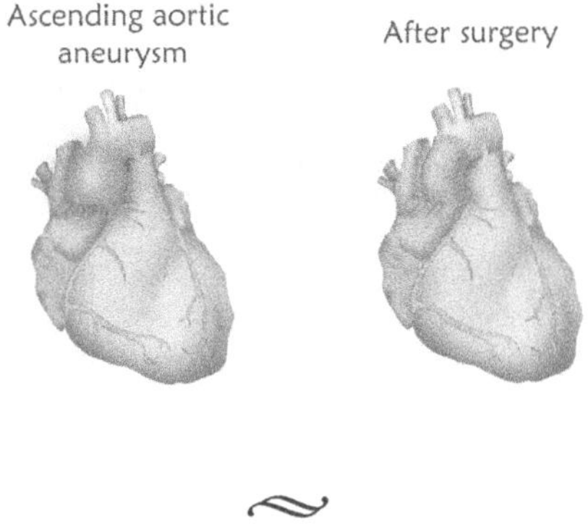

Aneurysm Repair: Surgical repair of an aneurysm typically involves replacing the weakened section of the artery with a synthetic graft.

Each of these procedures has its own risks and benefits, and the decision to proceed with surgery should involve a thorough discussion between the patient and a multidisciplinary team of healthcare providers, including a cardiac surgeon, a cardiologist, and a geneticist familiar with EDS.

Aneurysm treatment

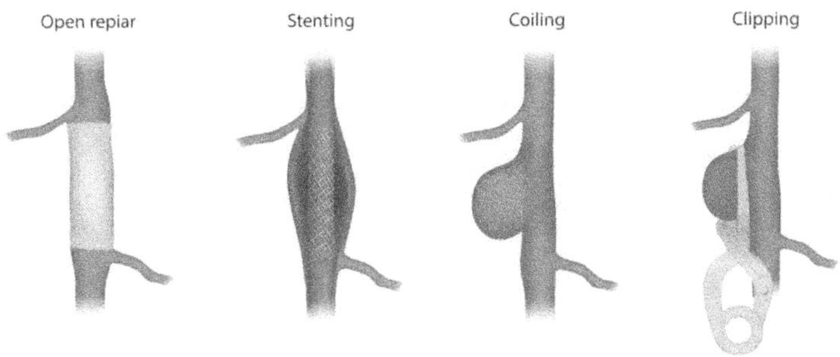

POSTOPERATIVE CARE

After cardiovascular surgery, patients with EDS require careful postoperative care and follow-up. Given the connective tissue abnormalities in EDS, postoperative healing can be challenging and complications may arise. Therefore, monitoring and management should be performed by a multidisciplinary team experienced in treating EDS.

Immediate Postoperative Care

In the immediate postoperative phase, the focus is on stabilizing the patient and managing pain. Patients are typically monitored in an intensive care unit (ICU) where vital signs, neurologic status, and wound healing can be closely observed.

Early Postoperative Care

Once stabilized, the patient is moved to a regular ward for further care. This phase focuses on:

- **Pain Management:** Adequate pain control is essential for recovery. Pain management strategies often involve a combination of medications, including opioids, non-steroidal anti-inflammatory drugs (NSAIDs), and adjunctive medications like gabapentin.
- **Wound Care:** Dressings are routinely changed and the surgical wound is closely monitored for signs of infection or poor healing, both of which can be more common in patients with EDS due to their abnormal connective tissue.
- **Mobilization:** Early mobilization is encouraged to prevent complications such as deep vein thrombosis (DVT) and to promote overall recovery.
- **Cardiac Rehabilitation:** Once the patient is medically stable, a structured cardiac rehabilitation program may begin. This involves carefully supervised exercise, education about heart-healthy living, and often, counseling to help the patient cope with the psychological aspects of their condition.

Long-Term Follow-Up

After discharge, long-term follow-up is crucial. This includes:

- **Regular Clinic Visits:** Patients will need to have regular follow-up appointments with their cardiac surgeon and cardiologist to monitor their recovery and any potential complications.

- **Imaging Studies:** Regular imaging studies, such as echocardiograms or CT scans, may be needed to monitor the status of the repaired or replaced structures and to check for new problems.
- **Lifestyle Modifications and Medication Management:** Patients may need to make lifestyle changes, such as adopting a heart-healthy diet, quitting smoking, and incorporating regular physical activity. They will also need to manage medications for pain, blood pressure, cholesterol, and possibly anticoagulation, depending on their individual situation.

Each patient's follow-up plan will be tailored to their individual needs, based on their specific type of surgery, overall health status, and the severity of their EDS symptoms.

GASTROINTESTINAL SURGERY

Abdominal surgery may be indicated in EDS patients for a variety of reasons, primarily when non-surgical treatments do not provide sufficient relief or in cases of emergency.

INDICATIONS

Gastrointestinal complications are common in EDS due to the connective tissue disorders affecting the digestive system. Issues can range from functional gastrointestinal disorders, such as irritable bowel syndrome (IBS), to more severe complications like intestinal or arterial rupture, which require immediate surgical intervention.

Indications for abdominal surgery in EDS patients may include:

<u>Gastrointestinal perforation or rupture:</u> Gastrointestinal perforation, while rare, is a severe and potentially life-threatening complication that can occur in individuals with certain types of EDS. This condition happens when a hole forms all the way through the stomach, small intestine, or large bowel. Due to the fragility and decreased integrity of the connective tissue in the gastrointestinal tract in EDS patients, they are at higher risk for such perforations. Symptoms can include severe abdominal pain, nausea, vomiting, and fever. It's considered a medical emergency and typically requires immediate surgery to repair the hole and prevent sepsis, a life-threatening infection that can spread throughout the body.

Gastrointestinal tract

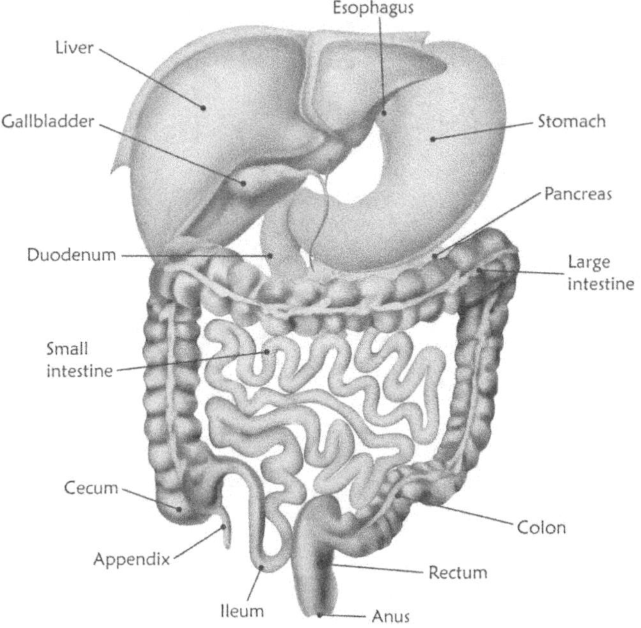

 Conditions like gastroparesis or chronic intestinal pseudo-obstruction, when they do not respond to other treatments, may necessitate surgical interventions such as the insertion of a feeding tube or even small bowel transplantation in extreme cases.

GASTROPARESIS

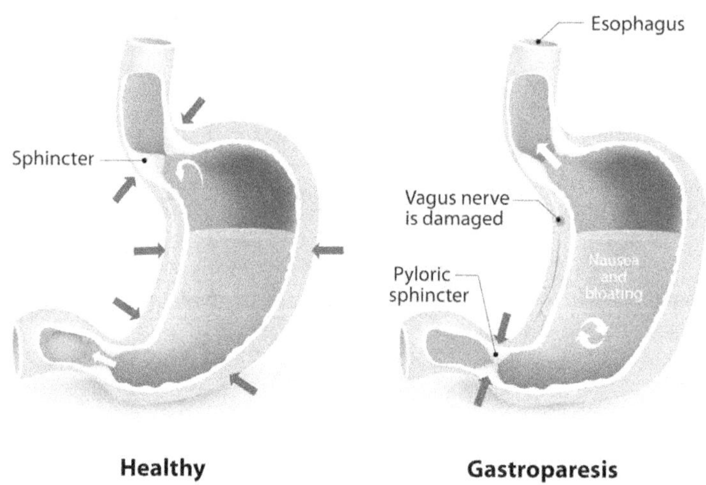

Hernias: One common complication of EDS is the development of hernias, particularly gastrointestinal hernias. A hernia occurs when an organ pushes through an opening in the muscle or tissue that holds it in place. In the case of gastrointestinal hernias, parts of the stomach or intestines protrude through a weakened area in the abdominal wall. Due to the inherent tissue fragility and elasticity in EDS, the abdominal wall can be more susceptible to developing such weaknesses. Symptoms can include pain, a noticeable bulge, and in severe cases, nausea, vomiting, and obstruction. Depending on the size and location of the hernia, treatment can range from watchful waiting to surgical intervention. As with all health concerns in EDS, management should be individualized, and care should be taken to address the underlying connective tissue disorder.

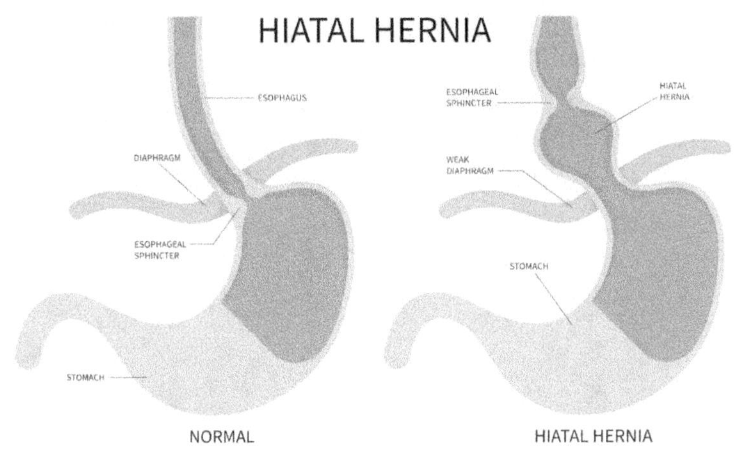

Severe or recurrent diverticulitis: Diverticulitis is an inflammation or infection of small pouches called diverticula that can develop along the walls of the digestive system. These pouches are more likely to form when the walls of the intestines are weak or under pressure, as can be the case with the connective tissue abnormalities seen in EDS. Symptoms of diverticulitis can include abdominal pain, fever, and changes in bowel habits. The management of diverticulitis in patients with EDS can be challenging due to the inherent fragility of the tissue, and it requires a personalized approach that often involves a combination of dietary modifications, medication, and in some severe cases, surgery.

Diverticulosis

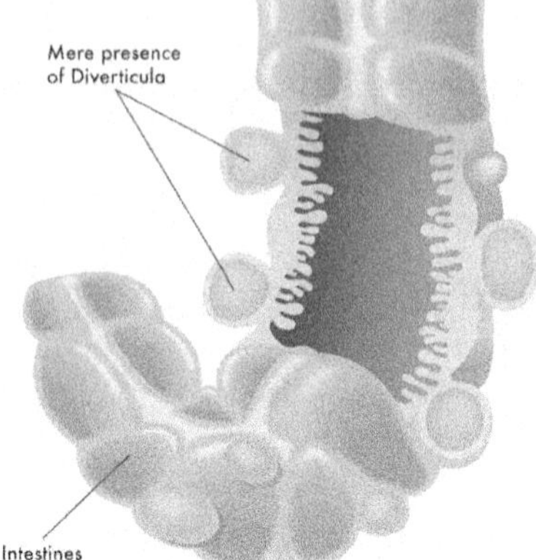

Diverticulitis

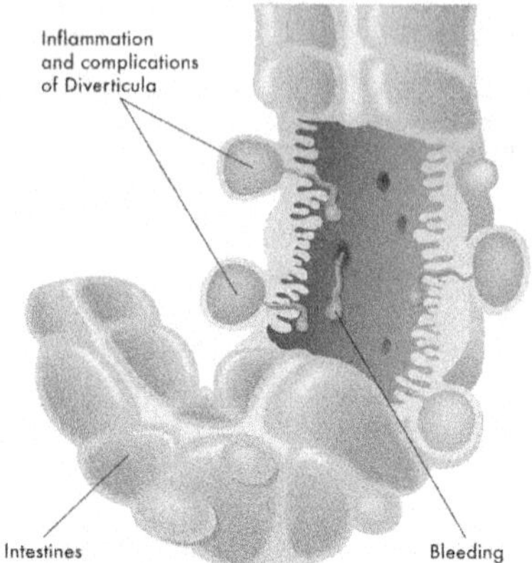

PROCEDURES

The type of surgical procedure performed depends on the specific condition and the individual patient's overall health and preference. Here are some procedures that might be considered:

<u>Laparoscopic surgery:</u> This is a minimally invasive surgery involving small incisions in the abdomen, through which a laparoscope (a long, thin tube with a high-intensity light and a high-resolution camera at the front) and surgical instruments are inserted. This technique could be used for various procedures, including hernia repair or removal of parts of the digestive tract.

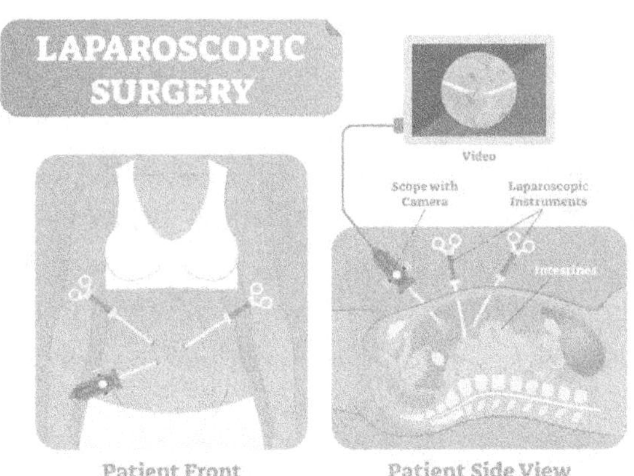

<u>**Open surgery:**</u> This involves a larger incision and is usually reserved for more complex cases or when laparoscopic surgery is not an option.

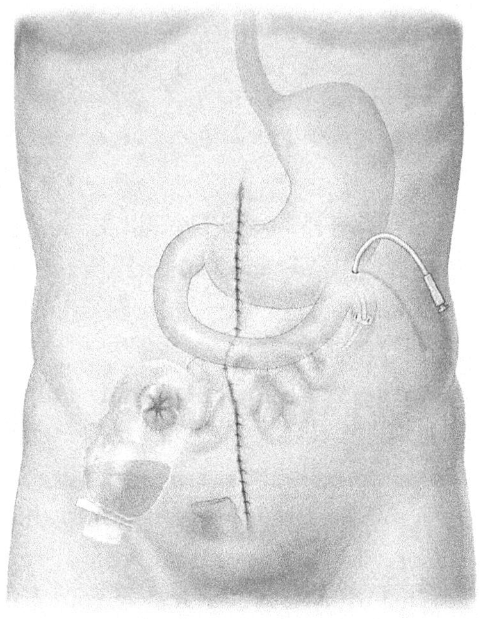

<u>**Feeding tube placement:**</u> In some cases, gastrointestinal involvement in EDS can lead to severe dysmotility, malnutrition, or the inability to eat enough food by mouth. For these patients, the placement of a feeding tube may be considered. A feeding tube is a medical device used to provide nutrition directly into the stomach or small intestine. This procedure, while beneficial, can present unique challenges in EDS patients due to their tissue fragility and healing complications. Therefore, careful consideration and planning are essential prior to the placement of feeding tubes. The choice of feeding tube

(nasogastric, gastrostomy, or jejunostomy) will depend on the individual's specific needs and overall health status.

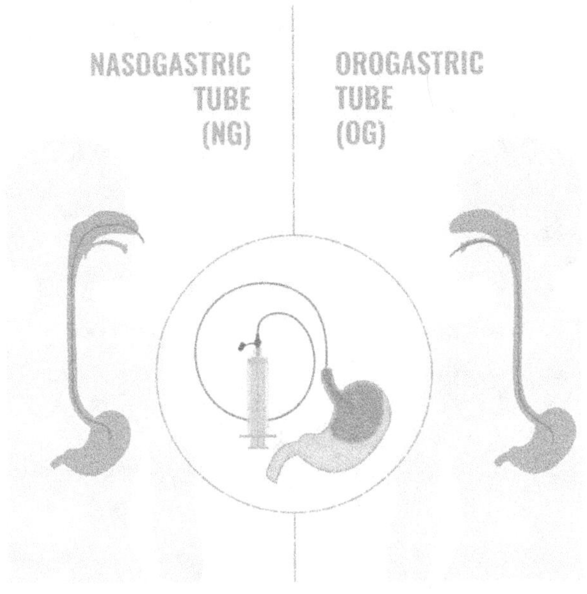

gastrostomy tube

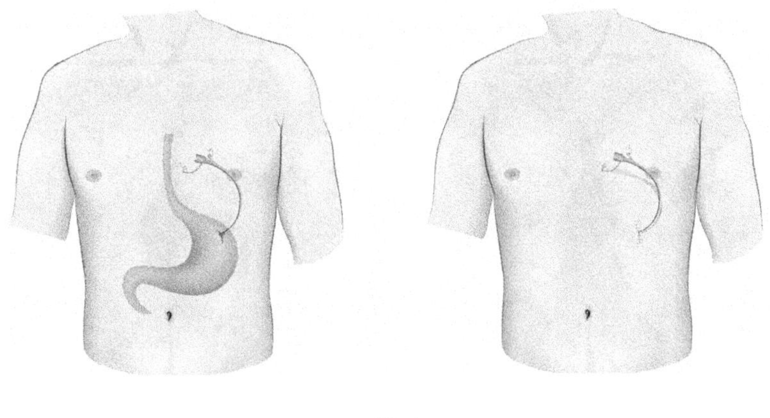

∼

Post-procedure care also requires close follow-up and coordination with a multidisciplinary team to manage potential complications like infection, dislodgement, or poor wound healing. Despite these challenges, a feeding tube can significantly improve the quality of life and nutritional status of EDS patients with severe gastrointestinal issues.

<u>Bowel resection:</u> In cases of recurrent diverticulitis or severe motility disorders, a section of the affected bowel may be removed.

TYPES OF OSTOMY

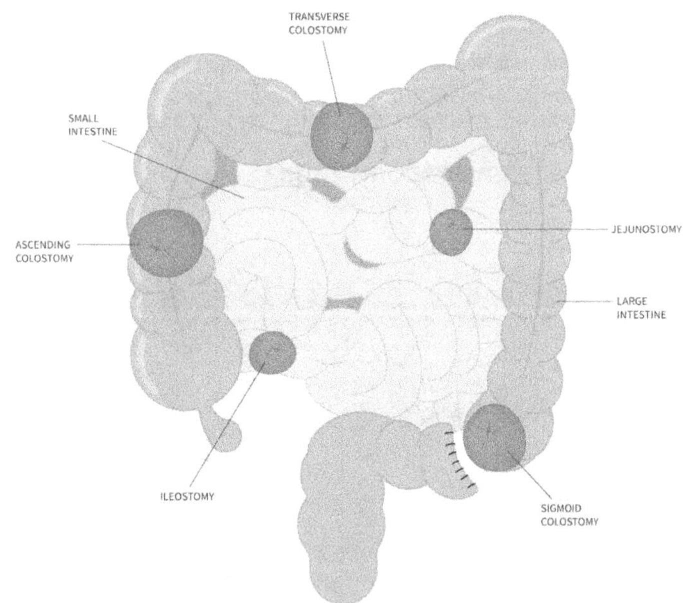

<u>Hernia repair:</u> This can be done laparoscopically or with open surgery, depending on the size and location of the hernia. It can pose unique challenges in surgical procedures like ventral hernia repair. A ventral hernia occurs when tissue bulges through an opening in the muscles of the abdomen. While the repair of these hernias is often straightforward in the general population, patients with EDS can face an increased risk of postoperative complications due to their underlying connective tissue abnormalities. Wound dehiscence (separation of the wound edges) is a particular concern, as the fragile and elastic skin can struggle to heal from the surgical incision. Post-surgical infections may also be more common in EDS patients. In some cases, the hernia may recur, as the weakened tissue struggles to hold the repair. Postoperative care for these patients should be carefully managed, with close monitoring for complications and strategies to support wound healing and tissue repair. Despite these challenges, with careful surgical planning and postoperative care, successful hernia repair is possible in patients with EDS.

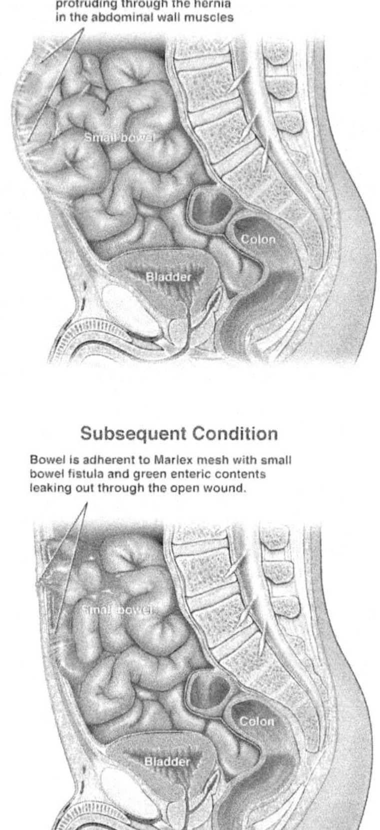

It's important to note that surgery in EDS patients requires careful consideration due to potential complications related to the syndrome, such as poor wound healing and increased bleeding. Therefore, surgical interventions are usually considered when other treatment options have been exhausted, or in the case of life-threatening emergencies.

After the procedure, patients may need a carefully planned recovery period, which often involves pain management, wound care, and physical therapy. The rehabilitation process is crucial to restore function and improve the quality of life after surgery.

As always, the decision to proceed with surgery should be made after thoughtful discussion and consideration of the risks and benefits, in consultation with knowledgeable and experienced healthcare providers. It should take into account the patient's unique situation, including their specific type of EDS, overall health, lifestyle, and personal preferences.

POSTOPERATIVE CARE

The care taken after gastrointestinal surgery plays a crucial role in the patient's recovery, particularly in individuals with EDS, who may face additional challenges due to their underlying condition. Here are some key components of postoperative care and follow-up:

IMMEDIATE POSTOPERATIVE CARE

This phase involves close monitoring of the patient in the post-anesthesia care unit (PACU) or intensive care unit (ICU), depending on the severity of the case. Vital signs, pain levels, and signs of any immediate complications such as bleeding, infection, or adverse reactions to anesthesia are closely observed.

Pain Management

Pain management is a critical aspect of postoperative care. An individualized pain management plan is typically designed, taking into consideration the nature of the surgery, the patient's overall health, and their personal tolerance to pain. This often involves a combination of medications, ranging from non-opioid analgesics (like acetaminophen and non-steroidal anti-inflammatory drugs) to opioids for more severe pain.

Wound Care

For patients with EDS, wound healing can be a significant challenge due to the nature of their skin and tissues. Special care must be taken to prevent infection and promote healing. This includes regular cleaning of the wound, careful dressing changes, and monitoring for signs of infection such as redness, swelling, increased pain, or discharge.

Nutrition Support

Given the impact of gastrointestinal surgery on digestion and absorption, nutritional support is crucial. Initially, patients may receive nutrition intravenously or through a feeding tube. As the patient recovers, they will gradually transition back to oral feeding, often starting with a liquid diet and slowly reintroducing solid foods. A dietitian may provide advice on suitable dietary choices to facilitate healing and overall health.

Physical Activity and Rehabilitation

Early mobilization is encouraged to promote circulation and prevent complications such as deep vein thrombosis (DVT). However, the extent and type of physical activity allowed will depend on the specific surgery. Physical therapists can provide guidance on safe and effective exercises to gradually restore strength and mobility.

Follow-up Appointments

Regular follow-up appointments with the surgeon and other members of the healthcare team are essential. These visits allow for the monitoring of the patient's recovery, addressing any concerns or complications, and adjusting the treatment plan as necessary.

Psychological Support

The postoperative period can be emotionally challenging. Psychological support, whether from a professional or a support network of family and friends, can help patients cope with the stress and anxiety that may accompany surgery and recovery.

LONG-TERM FOLLOW-UP

Given the chronic nature of EDS, long-term follow-up is crucial. This may involve ongoing management of EDS symptoms, monitoring for potential late complications related to the surgery, and adjustments to the patient's overall treatment plan.

Each patient's postoperative care plan will be individualized based on their speci!c circumstances, including the type of EDS, the nature of the surgery, and their overall health status.

EYE SURGERY

EDS is a collection of inherited disorders affecting the body's connective tissues. These abnormalities can also lead to various ocular problems, as the eye is rich in connective tissue. **Keratoconus**, a progressive eye disease in which the normally round cornea thins and begins to bulge into a cone-like shape, is more common in individuals with EDS. This can lead to visual distortion and myopia.

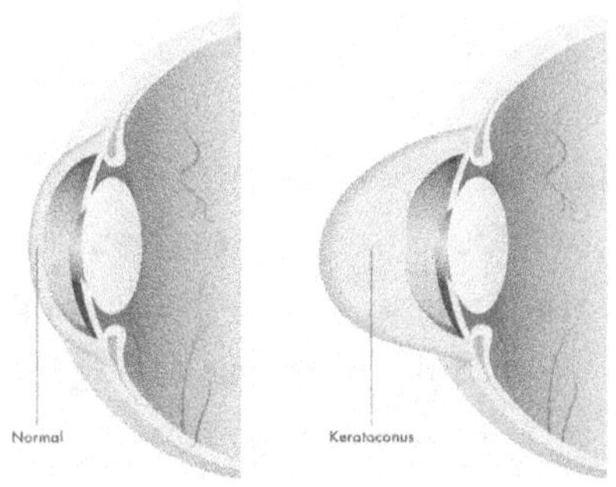

Blue sclera, where the whites of the eyes have a bluish hue due to the thinness of the sclera, is another common feature.

EDS patients may also experience retinal detachment, a serious condition where the retina pulls away from its normal position at the back of the eye, leading to potential vision loss.

Other potential issues include early-onset **glaucoma**, a disease that damages the eye's optic nerve, and dry eyes. Therefore, regular eye examinations are essential for individuals with EDS to monitor and manage these potential complications.

COMMON OCULAR CONDITIONS IN EDS

Dry eyes: Dry eye syndrome, characterized by the eyes' inability to stay adequately lubricated, is one of the ocular manifestations that individuals with EDS can experience. Symptoms can include a burning or stinging sensation in the eyes, a gritty or sandy feeling as if something is in the eye, redness, sensitivity to light, and blurred vision. These symptoms can fluctuate throughout the day and can be influenced by environmental factors such as wind, dry air, or prolonged screen time.

The cause of dry eyes in EDS patients can be multifactorial. It may be due to an underlying dysfunction in the tear-producing glands, which could be directly related to the connective tissue abnormalities seen in EDS.

Certain medications and the long-term use of contact lenses can also contribute to dry eyes. Non-surgical treatment options are the primary approach to managing dry eyes in EDS patients. Over-the-counter artificial tear solutions are often the first line of treatment, providing temporary relief by supplementing natural tear production.

Lubricating eye ointments can provide longer-lasting relief, especially overnight. In some cases, medications may be prescribed to reduce inflammation around the tear glands or increase tear production. Lifestyle changes, such as taking frequent breaks during computer work, protecting the eyes from wind and dry air, and staying well-hydrated, can also help manage symptoms. In more severe cases, an eye care professional may recommend procedures such as punctal plugs, which involve blocking the tear ducts to retain more natural tears on the eye's surface.

Myopia and astigmatism: Myopia is characterized by difficulty seeing objects at a distance while close-up vision remains clear.

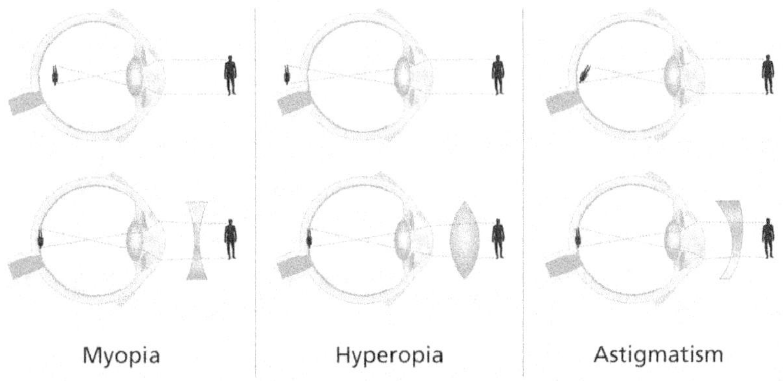

In people with EDS, myopia could be due to elongation of the eyeball or changes in the shape of the cornea or lens, which are rich in connective tissue. Astigmatism, on the other hand, is caused by an irregularly shaped cornea or lens that prevents light from focusing properly on the retina, leading to blurred or distorted vision at all distances.

Non-surgical treatment options for both myopia and astigmatism primarily involve correcting the refractive error with glasses or contact lenses. Glasses are often the first line of treatment, and they work by redirecting light onto the correct part of the retina. Contact lenses perform a similar function but are placed directly on the surface of the eye. For individuals with EDS who may have more sensitive eyes or problems with dry eye syndrome, special care is needed in the fitting and selection of contact lenses to ensure comfort.

Another non-surgical option is orthokeratology (Ortho-K), a treatment that involves wearing rigid gas-permeable contact lenses overnight to reshape the cornea temporarily, thus improving vision during the day. However, it should be noted that the effects of Ortho-K are temporary, and discontinuation of lens wear leads to the return of the original refractive error. - Retinal detachment: symptoms, causes, and urgency of surgical intervention

EYE SURGERIES RELEVANT TO EDS PATIENTS

The primary indications for eye surgeries in patients with EDS are the treatment of severe refractive errors (like high myopia and astigmatism), retinal detachments, and keratoconus. In the case of significant refractive errors that are not adequately managed with glasses or contact lenses, refractive surgeries such as LASIK or PRK might be considered. However, the decision to proceed with these surgeries must be taken carefully due to potential issues with wound healing and increased risk of corneal ectasia (a bulging of the cornea) post-surgery in EDS patients.

For retinal detachments, which can occur more frequently in EDS due to the fragility of the connective tissue supporting the retina, surgical intervention is necessary to reattach the retina and prevent permanent vision loss. Vitrectomy and scleral buckle are common surgical procedures used in these cases. Keratoconus, a condition causing the cornea to thin and bulge outwards, is another ocular issue associated with EDS. If the disease progresses to a severe stage, corneal cross-linking or even corneal transplant may be required.

<u>LASIK and PRK:</u> LASIK (Laser-Assisted In Situ Keratomileusis) and PRK (Photorefractive Keratectomy) are two common types of refractive eye surgery used to correct vision problems such as myopia (nearsightedness), hyperopia (farsightedness), and astigmatism. Both procedures aim to reshape the cornea, the clear front surface of the eye, allowing light entering the eye to be properly focused onto the retina for clear vision.

LASIK involves creating a thin flap on the cornea's surface, lifting it, and then using a laser to remove a precise amount of corneal tissue underneath. The flap is then replaced, which aids in the healing process.

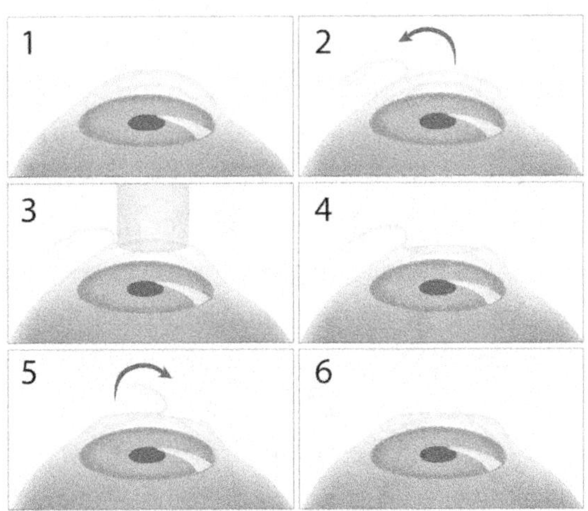

Lasik Eye Surgery

In contrast, **PRK** does not involve creating a flap. Instead, the outer layer of the cornea (epithelium) is removed, and the laser is applied to the exposed corneal tissue. The epithelium regrows over the treated area in the days following the procedure.

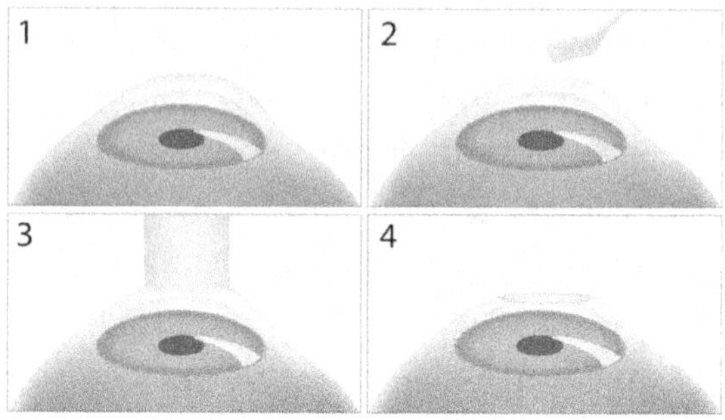

Photorefractive Keratectomy (PRK)

For patients with EDS, considerations need to be taken before opting for LASIK or PRK. EDS is characterized by abnormalities in the connective tissue, and since the cornea is rich in connective tissue, there may be potential complications. For instance, EDS patients might face a higher risk of corneal ectasia, a thinning and bulging of the corneal tissue, after LASIK. Also, slower wound healing, a common issue in EDS, might impact the recovery process after surgery. Therefore, while LASIK and PRK can be effective in treating refractive errors, they should be considered carefully in patients with EDS, and a thorough discussion with the eye care professional is essential before making a decision.

Cataract surgery: Cataract surgery is a procedure that removes the lens of your eye when it has become cloudy and impairs your vision, a condition known as a cataract. During the surgery, the cloudy lens is removed and is usually replaced with an artificial lens, called an intraocular lens (IOL). The IOL becomes a permanent part of your eye and functions much like your natural lens. Cataract surgery is a common and generally safe procedure that can significantly improve visual acuity and quality of life.

While cataracts are often related to aging, they can also occur due to other factors such as prolonged use of certain medications, exposure to UV radiation, or underlying health conditions like diabetes. People with EDS may also be prone to early-onset cataracts, although the correlation is not fully understood. Symptoms of cataracts include blurred or double vision, sensitivity to light, and difficulty seeing at night.

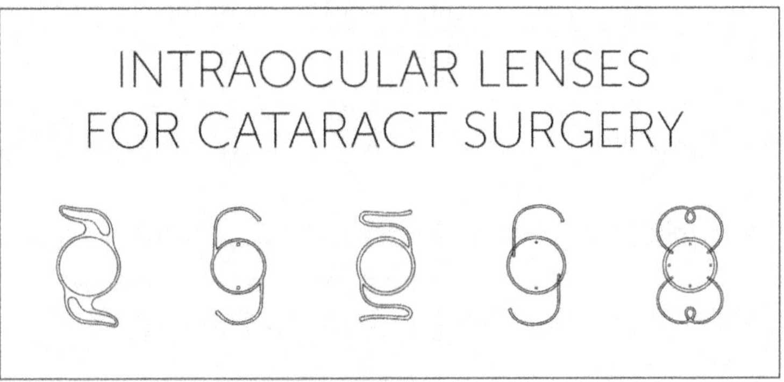

For patients with EDS, it's important to remember that the potential complications make preoperative planning and post-operative care crucial. Surgeons might need to consider using special techniques or adjustments during the surgery to accommodate the patient's unique needs.

Corneal transplant: A corneal transplant, also known as keratoplasty, is a surgical procedure where a damaged or diseased cornea is replaced with healthy corneal tissue from a donor. There are different types of corneal transplants, including full-thickness (penetrating keratoplasty) and partial-thickness (lamellar keratoplasty) transplants. The procedure can help restore vision, reduce pain, and improve the appearance of a damaged or diseased cornea.

One of the common reasons for a corneal transplant is keratoconus, a condition where the cornea, which is typically round, bulges into a cone-like shape due to thinning. This distortion of the cornea leads to progressive vision impairment that may not be adequately corrected with glasses or contact lenses. In advanced stages or when corneal scarring occurs, a corneal transplant may be required to restore vision.

For patients with EDS, corneal transplantation needs to be considered carefully. EDS is characterized by defects in the connective tissue, which can affect the cornea and potentially lead to complications such as increased risk of graft failure or graft rejection. Moreover, EDS patients often have slower wound healing, which might affect the recovery process after the surgery. Therefore, while a corneal transplant can be a viable solution for severe keratoconus or other corneal diseases, it is crucial that patients with EDS have a thorough discussion with their eye care professional about the potential benefits and risks before making a decision.

<u>Scleral buckle or vitrectomy for retinal detachment:</u> Scleral buckle and vitrectomy are two surgical procedures commonly used in the treatment of retinal detachment, a serious condition where the retina, which is the light-sensitive layer at the back of the eye, separates from the underlying tissue. Without prompt treatment, retinal detachment can lead to permanent vision loss.

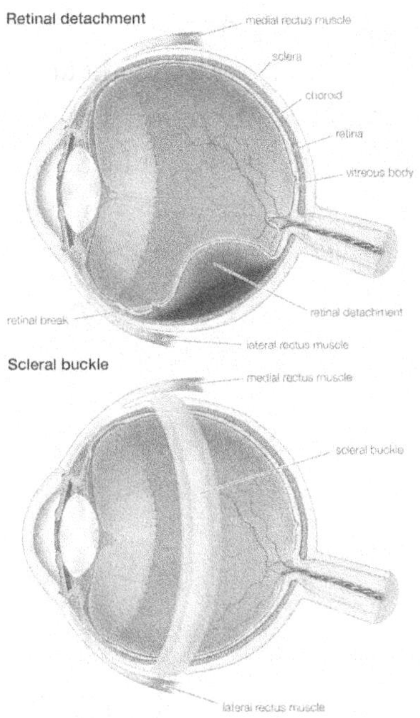

A scleral buckle involves placing a flexible band (the buckle) around the eye to counteract the force pulling the retina out of place, thereby allowing the retina to reattach. On the other hand, a vitrectomy involves removing the vitreous, a gel-like substance that fills the eye, to prevent it from pulling on the retina.

Once the vitreous is removed, it is replaced with a gas or silicone oil to help the retina reattach. These procedures are often successful in reattaching the retina and preventing further vision loss.

Patients with EDS might be at an increased risk for retinal detachment due to the fragility of their connective tissue. While these surgeries can be effective, EDS patients may face unique challenges due to their condition. For instance, slower wound healing and increased risk of infection are considerations with EDS, which might impact the recovery process.

Additionally, the sclera (white of the eye) may be more prone to thinning in EDS patients, which could affect the outcome of a scleral buckle procedure. Therefore, the decision to proceed with either of these surgeries should be made after a thorough discussion between the patient and their eye care professional about the potential risks and benefits.

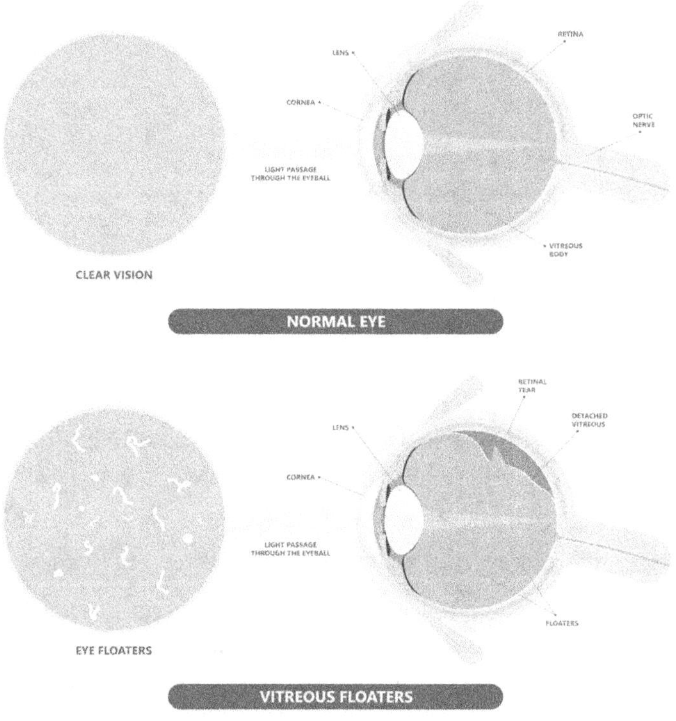

PSYCHOLOGICAL SUPPORT

THE PSYCHOSOCIAL IMPACT OF EDS

EDS, while primarily a physical condition, has far-reaching effects on a person's mental and social health. The wide array of symptoms and their unpredictable nature can create a life of uncertainty for those living with the syndrome. These symptoms can range from mild to debilitating, with some individuals experiencing life-threatening complications. This unpredictability often leads to heightened anxiety and stress levels, impacting the overall quality of life.

The emotional and psychological impact of EDS cannot be overstated. Chronic illnesses like EDS often lead to feelings of anxiety and depression. The unpredictability of symptom flare-ups can create a life of uncertainty, leading to heightened stress levels. Moreover, the continuous need to manage and adapt to a changing array of symptoms can lead to emotional exhaustion. The constant pain and discomfort, coupled with the lack of understanding from others, can also lead to feelings of isolation and loneliness. Recognizing and addressing these mental health challenges is a crucial part of managing EDS.

THE ROLE OF FAMILY AND SOCIAL SUPPORT NETWORKS

Family and social support networks play a critical role in managing the psychosocial impact of EDS. The support of loved ones can provide emotional relief, practical help, and a sense of understanding and acceptance that is often lacking elsewhere. Social support networks, including support groups and online communities, can provide a platform for patients to share their experiences, learn from others, and gain a sense of belonging. These networks can also play a crucial role in educating others about EDS and advocating for patient needs.

COPING MECHANISMS AND THERAPIES FOR EDS PATIENTS

Coping with the psychosocial impact of EDS requires a combination of strategies. Psychological therapies, such as cognitive-behavioral therapy (CBT) and mindfulness-based stress reduction (MBSR), have shown promise in helping individuals manage chronic pain, anxiety, and depression associated with EDS. Physical therapies and regular exercise, tailored to the individual's abilities, can help manage physical symptoms and improve overall well-being. Additionally, finding healthy ways to express emotions, such as through art or writing, can provide emotional relief and a sense of control over one's experiences.

THE ROLE OF PSYCHOLOGICAL SUPPORT

Given these challenges, psychological support becomes a crucial component of managing EDS. Providing holistic care that encompasses both physical and mental health can greatly improve the quality of life of people with EDS. Psychological support can be delivered in various ways. Here are some key elements:

Cognitive Behavioral Therapy (CBT)

Cognitive Behavioral Therapy (CBT) is a form of psychotherapy that has proven effective in managing a range of emotional and psychological challenges, including those associated with chronic illnesses like EDS. The fundamental premise of CBT is that our thoughts, feelings, and behaviors are interconnected, and by modifying maladaptive thoughts and behaviors, we can alter our emotional responses and overall well-being.

For EDS patients, CBT can be a game-changer. Living with a chronic illness often leads to a cycle of negative thoughts and emotions, which can exacerbate physical symptoms and create a vicious circle of distress. For instance, a patient might have the thought, "I can't do anything right because of my condition," leading to feelings of worthlessness and depression, which might then lead to withdrawal from activities and worsening of physical symptoms.

CBT helps break this cycle by teaching patients to identify and challenge these negative thought patterns and replace them with more accurate and constructive ones. For example, the thought, "I can't do anything right because of my condition," might be replaced with, "EDS makes certain activities more challenging, but there are still many things I can do well and enjoy."

Moreover, CBT can also equip EDS patients with effective coping mechanisms for managing pain and fatigue, such as relaxation techniques, pacing strategies, and problem-solving skills. By enhancing patients' self-efficacy and control over their symptoms, CBT can significantly improve the quality of life for EDS patients.

It's important to note, however, that the effectiveness of CBT can vary from person to person, and it is not a cure for EDS or its physical symptoms. But it can be a powerful tool in the broader toolkit of managing the psychosocial impact of EDS.

Support Groups

Support groups can play a vital role in managing the psychosocial impact of living with EDS. These groups provide a safe space for patients to connect with others who are going through similar experiences, offering a sense of understanding and camaraderie that can be hard to find elsewhere.

Support groups can provide a platform for sharing

personal experiences, tips, and strategies for managing the physical and psychosocial challenges of EDS. They can also serve as a source of up-to-date information about the condition and new treatments or therapies that may be beneficial.

The value of shared experiences in support groups cannot be overstated. Understanding that there are others who are going through similar challenges can alleviate feelings of isolation and loneliness that often accompany chronic illnesses like EDS. It can also instill a sense of hope, as members witness others successfully managing their symptoms and leading fulfilling lives despite the challenges.

Furthermore, support groups often foster a sense of empowerment among their members. They can provide opportunities for advocacy, enabling members to raise awareness about EDS and contribute to a greater understanding and acceptance of the condition in the wider community.

Support groups can take many forms, from in-person meetings to online communities. Online support groups, in particular, have become increasingly popular due to their accessibility and the anonymity they can provide, making them a good option for individuals who may have mobility challenges or feel uncomfortable discussing their experiences in person.

It's important to note that while support groups provide valuable emotional support and community, they are not a substitute for professional medical advice. Members should always consult with healthcare professionals for the management of EDS and any associated symptoms.

Individual Counseling

Individual counseling is another key tool in managing the psychosocial impact of EDS. Unlike group therapy or support groups, individual counseling offers a one-on-one environment where patients can explore their feelings, fears, and challenges in a confidential and non-judgmental setting.

Counseling can provide a space for patients to express their thoughts and emotions related to their condition that they might not feel comfortable sharing with others. It allows for deep, personalized exploration of the effects of EDS on the individual's life, including their relationships, self-esteem, and mental health.

One of the primary benefits of individual counseling is its adaptability to the unique needs of the patient. Each person's experience with EDS is different, and individual counseling allows for a personalized approach that takes into account the patient's specific symptoms, lifestyle, and emotional state. This personalized approach can lead to more targeted and effective strategies for managing the psychosocial impact of EDS.

Counseling for EDS patients often involves elements of cognitive-behavioral therapy (CBT), focusing on identifying and challenging negative thought patterns, as well as developing coping strategies for managing chronic pain and other physical symptoms. However, it can also incorporate other therapeutic approaches, such as mindfulness-based therapies, trauma-informed therapies, or acceptance and commitment therapy (ACT), depending on the patient's needs and preferences.

In addition to emotional and psychological support, counselors can also provide practical assistance, such as helping patients navigate the healthcare system, advocating for accommodations in the workplace or school, and providing guidance on communicating effectively with healthcare professionals, family members, and friends about their condition.

. . .

Family Therapy

Family therapy can be an essential part of managing the psychosocial impact of EDS. EDS affects not just the individual diagnosed with the syndrome, but also their family members who may struggle to understand the condition and how to provide the best support. Family therapy provides a platform for families to explore these issues together and foster stronger, more supportive relationships.

Family therapy can help family members better understand EDS and its impact on the patient's day-to-day life. Through therapy, families can learn about the unpredictability of symptom flare-ups, the invisible nature of some symptoms, and the emotional toll of living with a chronic condition. This increased understanding can lead to greater empathy and improved communication within the family.

In addition, family therapy can provide families with strategies to manage the challenges that come with EDS. This can include practical strategies for managing physical symptoms, as well as emotional support strategies. For example, family members can learn how to provide emotional support during symptom flare-ups, how to handle their own feelings of stress or helplessness, and how to foster a positive and supportive home environment.

Family therapy can also help address any feelings of guilt, resentment, or frustration that may arise within the family due to the challenges of EDS. These feelings are common, especially among siblings who may feel that their needs are being overshadowed by the needs of the family member with EDS. Family therapy can help validate these feelings and provide strategies to manage them in a way that supports the well-being of all family members.

It's important to note that family therapy should be conducted by a therapist who is knowledgeable about EDS to ensure that the therapy is informed and beneficial. Overall, family therapy can be a powerful tool in managing the psychosocial impact of EDS, fostering understanding, empathy, and support within the family.

Mindfulness and Relaxation Techniques

Mindfulness and relaxation techniques can be highly beneficial for individuals with EDS. These practices can help manage stress, reduce pain, improve sleep, and enhance overall well-being.

Mindfulness

Mindfulness involves focusing one's awareness on the present moment, calmly acknowledging and accepting one's feelings, thoughts, and bodily sensations. For EDS patients, mindfulness can be a valuable tool in managing both the physical and emotional challenges associated with the condition.

Practicing mindfulness can help EDS patients better understand their pain and other physical sensations, rather than trying to avoid or suppress them. This awareness can lead to a more nuanced understanding of their bodies, enabling a more proactive and effective management of symptoms.

In an emotional context, mindfulness can help patients manage the stress, anxiety, and depression that often accompany chronic illnesses like EDS. By learning to accept and sit with their emotions without judgment, EDS patients can reduce the intensity of negative feelings and increase their emotional resilience.

Relaxation Techniques

Relaxation techniques, such as deep breathing, progressive muscle relaxation, guided imagery, and yoga, can also be beneficial for EDS patients. These practices can induce the body's relaxation response, a state of rest that can counteract the stress response.

Relaxation techniques can help reduce chronic pain, a common symptom of EDS, by relaxing tense muscles and lowering overall tension in the body. They can also improve sleep, another common issue for EDS patients, by promoting physical and mental relaxation at bedtime.

Moreover, regular practice of relaxation techniques can lower stress levels over time, leading to better emotional well-being and a higher quality of life.

SUPPLEMENTARY

BEIGHTON SCORE

The Beighton Score and the Five-Point Questionnaire are diagnostic tools used to assess joint hypermobility, a common symptom in conditions like EDS and other connective tissue disorders.

BEIGHTON SCORE

The Beighton Score is a simple, nine-point system used to evaluate joint hypermobility. A higher score indicates a greater degree of hypermobility. The test involves five maneuvers, four of which are done bilaterally:

1. Forward bending to place palms on the ground with straight legs (1 point).
2. Hyperextension of the knees beyond 10 degrees (1 point for each knee).
3. Hyperextension of the elbows beyond 10 degrees (1 point for each elbow).
4. Passive dorsiflexion of the little fingers beyond 90 degrees (1 point for each hand).
5. Passive apposition of the thumbs to the flexor aspects of the forearm (1 point for each thumb).

A score of 4 or more is typically considered indicative of joint hypermobility.

FIVE-POINT QUESTIONNAIRE

The Five-Point Questionnaire, also known as the Five-Point Hypermobility Questionnaire, is another tool used to assess hypermobility. It consists of five yes-or-no questions:

1. Can you now (or could you ever) place your hands flat on the floor without bending your knees?
2. Can you now (or could you ever) bend your thumb to touch your forearm?
3. As a child, did you amuse your friends by contorting your body into strange shapes or could you do the splits?
4. As a child or teenager, did your shoulder or kneecap dislocate on more than one occasion?
5. Do you consider yourself double-jointed?

Each "yes" answer is given 1 point. A score of 2 or more is typically used as a cut-off for identifying joint hypermobility.

Both of these tools are helpful for doctors when evaluating

potential cases of EDS or other connective tissue disorders, but they are not definitive diagnostic tests. Other factors, such as a complete medical history and additional physical examination findings, are also considered in the diagnostic process.

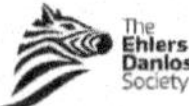

THE BEIGHTON SCORING SYSTEM
Measuring joint hypermobility

A. 5th FINGER / 'PINKIES'

Test **both sides**. Rest palm of the hand and forearm a **flat surface** with palm side down and fingers out straight.

Can the **fifth finger** be bent/lifted upwards at the knuckle to go back **beyond 90 degrees?**

If yes, add **one point** for each hand.

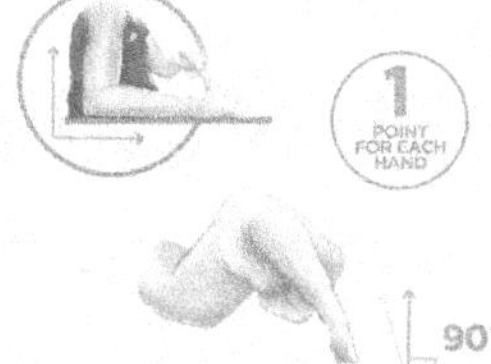

B. THUMBS

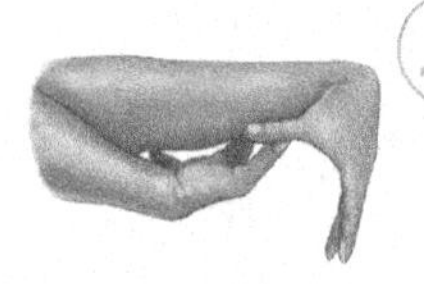

Test **both sides**: With the arm out straight, the palm facing down, and the wrist then fully bent downward, can the thumb be pushed back to touch the forearm?

If yes, add **one point** for each thumb.

C. ELBOWS

Test **both sides**: With arms outstretched and palms facing upwards, does the elbow extend (bend too far) upwards **more than an extra 10 degrees** beyond a normal outstretched position?

If yes, add **one point** for each side.

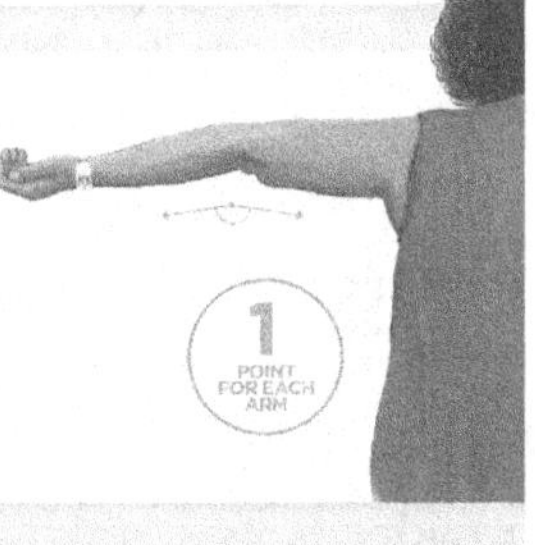

D. KNEES

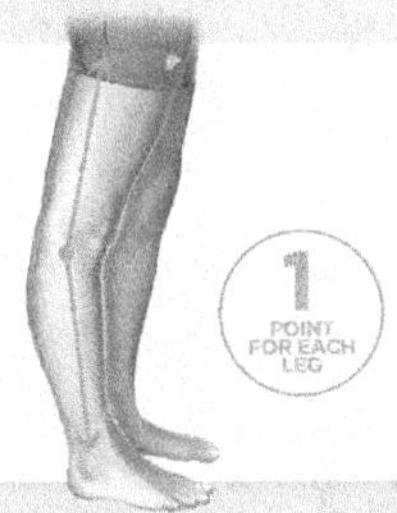

Test **both sides**: While standing, with knees locked (bent backwards as far as possible), does the lower part of either leg extend **more than 10 degrees forward?**

If yes, add **one point** for each side.

E. SPINE

Bend forward, can you place the palms of your hands **flat on the floor in front of your feet without bending your knees?**

If yes, **add one point.**

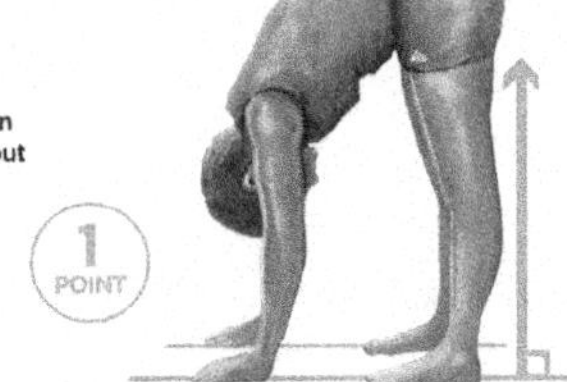

STRENGTHENING EXERCISES

This section is designed to help readers supplement their existing fitness regimen, promote muscle endurance, and provide a fresh approach to strength training. The exercises can be performed almost anywhere, with minimal or no equipment, making it easy to incorporate them into any lifestyle.

As always, we recommend that readers consult with a healthcare provider before starting any new exercise regimen. It's important to ensure all exercises are performed with the correct form to prevent any injuries.

For visual guidance on how to correctly perform these exercises, readers should search for each exercise by name on the internet or refer to reputable fitness resources. These videos can also be found at: https://rumble.com/c/c-3469560

OVERVIEW

The following table provides a comprehensive selection of 10 isometric exercises that target various muscle groups. Each exercise is listed along with the primary muscles it targets and the recommended number of repetitions per day and per week. Isometric exercises are a type of strength training where the joint angle and muscle length do not change during contraction. They're performed in static positions, rather than being dynamic through a range of motion.

Exercise Name	Targeted Muscles	Repetitions (per day)
Wall Sit	Thighs, glutes	3 x 30 seconds
Isometric Push-up	Chest, triceps	3 x 15 seconds
Isometric Squat	Quads, Hamstrings, Glutes	3 x 30 seconds
Isometric Bicep Curl	Biceps	3 x 15 seconds
Plank	Abdominals, Lower back	3 x 30 seconds
Isometric Shoulder Hold	Deltoids	3 x 30 seconds
Isometric Calf Raise	Calves	3 x 30 seconds
Isometric Tricep Extension	Triceps	3 x 15 seconds
Isometric Neck Exercise	Neck muscles	3 x 15 seconds
Isometric Lunge	Quads, glutes	3 x 30 seconds per leg

HOW TO PERFORM THESE EXERCISES

1. **Plank:** Lie face down, then lift your body off the ground, supporting your weight on your forearms and toes. Your body should form a straight line from head to heels. Hold this position.
2. **Wall Sit:** Stand against a wall with your back flat against it. Slide down until your thighs are parallel to the floor, as if sitting in an invisible chair. Keep your back flat against the wall. Hold this position.
3. **Isometric Push-up:** Start in a high plank position. Lower your body as if you're doing a push-up, but stop when your chest is halfway to the floor. Hold this position.
4. **Isometric Squat:** Stand with your feet hip-width apart. Lower your body as if sitting back into a chair until your thighs are parallel to the floor. Hold this position.
5. **Isometric Bicep Curl:** Hold a weight with your arm bent at a 90-degree angle as if in the middle of a bicep curl. Hold this position.

6. **Isometric Shoulder Hold:** Stand with your feet shoulder-width apart. Hold a dumbbell in each hand and raise your arms to shoulder height. Keep your palms facing down. Hold this position.

7. **Isometric Calf Raise:** Stand upright and push through the balls of both feet to raise your body upward. Keep your abdominal muscles pulled in so that you move straight upward, not leaning forward or backward.

8. **Isometric Tricep Extension:** Stand with a dumbbell in your hand. Raise your arm above your head, then lower the weight behind your head by bending at the elbow. Hold when your elbow is at a 90-degree angle.

9. **Isometric Neck Exercise:** Sit or stand with good posture. Place your hand on your forehead and push your head into your hand without letting your head move forward. Hold this position.

10. **Isometric Lunge:** Step forward with one foot until your leg reaches a 90-degree angle. Your rear knee should remain parallel to the ground and your front knee shouldn't go beyond your toes. Hold this position then switch legs.

RANGE OF MOTION EXERCISES

OVERVIEW

Range of Motion (ROM) exercises are physical activities designed to maintain, improve, or restore the amount of movement possible at a joint. These exercises help to keep the joints flexible and functional by moving the joint through its full available range.

ROM exercises can be performed on all joints in the body, including the neck, shoulders, elbows, wrists, hips, knees, and ankles. They can be done in a variety of positions such as standing, sitting, or lying down, and often involve simple movements like bending, straightening, rotating, or stretching the joint.

These exercises are particularly beneficial for individuals who have joint stiffness or mobility issues due to conditions like arthritis, stroke, or after a surgical procedure. They can also be used as part of a warm-up routine for athletes or as a preventive measure to maintain joint health in older adults.

It's important to perform ROM exercises under the guidance of a healthcare professional or trained fitness instructor to ensure they are done correctly and safely. The frequency, intensity, and duration of these exercises can be tailored to meet an individual's speci!c needs and health status.

Name of the Exercise	Targeted Muscles	Repetitions Per Day
Shoulder Rolls	Trapezius, Deltoids	10
Neck Side Stretch	Sternocleidomastoid, Trapezius	10
Wrist Flexion/Extension	Forearm Flexors, Forearm Extensors	10
Ankle Circles	Tibialis Anterior, Gastrocnemius, Soleus	10
Hip Circles	Gluteus Maximus, Hip Flexors, Adductors, Abductors	10
Knee to Chest Stretch	Gluteus Maximus, Hamstrings	10
Arm Circles	Deltoids, Trapezius, Pectorals, Rhomboids	10
Leg Extensions	Quadriceps	10
Heel to Butt Stretch	Quadriceps	10
Seated Hamstring Stretch	Hamstrings	10

HOW TO PERFORM THESE EXERCISES

1. Shoulder Rolls: Stand or sit upright. Lift your shoulders up towards your ears, then roll them back and down. Repeat in the opposite direction: down, forward, and up.

2. Neck Side Stretch: Stand or sit upright. Tilt your head to one side, trying to touch your ear to your shoulder. Hold for a few seconds, then repeat on the other side.

3. Wrist Flexion/Extension: Extend your arm in front of you with your palm facing down. Gently bend your wrist up and down, holding for a few seconds in each position.

4. Ankle Circles: Sit or lie down and extend your leg. Rotate your ankle in a circular motion, then repeat in the opposite direction.

5. Hip Circles: Stand with your feet hip-width apart. Place your hands on your hips, and make circles with your hips, first in one direction, then in the other.

6. Knee to Chest Stretch: Lie on your back with your legs extended. Bring one knee up to your chest, holding it with your hands. Hold for a few seconds then switch to the other leg.

7. Arm Circles: Stand with your feet shoulder-width apart.

Extend your arms out to the sides at shoulder height. Make small circles with your arms, first in one direction, then in the other.

8. Leg Extensions: Sit in a chair with your feet flat on the floor. Extend one leg out in front of you, hold for a few seconds, then lower it back down. Repeat with the other leg.

9. Heel to Butt Stretch: Stand upright and balance on one leg. Bend your other knee, bringing your heel towards your buttocks. Hold your ankle with your hand to increase the stretch.

10. Seated Hamstring Stretch: Sit on the ground with one leg extended in front of you and the other bent with your foot against your thigh. Lean forward from your hips (try to keep your back straight) towards the foot of your extended leg. Hold for a few seconds, then switch legs.

Remember to always warm up before performing these exercises and cool down afterwards. Also, these exercises should never cause pain. If you feel pain, stop the exercise and consult with a healthcare professional.

PROPRIOCEPTIVE TRAINING

OVERVIEW

Proprioceptive training, also known as balance or stability training, is a type of exercise that improves your ability to sense the position, location, orientation, and movement of your body and its parts. This type of training is crucial for athletes, older adults, and people undergoing rehabilitation after injuries, as it improves coordination, reduces risk of injury, and aids in recovery.

Proprioceptive exercises often involve movements that challenge balance and stability, forcing the body to respond by adjusting its position. This not only helps improve balance and coordination but also strengthens key muscles and joints, thus enhancing overall physical performance.

The exercises range from simple tasks like standing on one leg, to more complex activities that require specialized equipment like stability balls, BOSU balls, or wobble boards. They can be incorporated into a regular workout routine or performed as a separate session.

The exercises often involve the lower body, as the legs and feet provide much of the feedback used in proprioception.

However, upper body and core muscles can also be involved, especially in exercises that require maintaining balance while moving or lifting weights.

It's important to perform proprioceptive exercises under the guidance of a healthcare professional or trained fitness instructor to ensure they are done correctly and safely. As with any form of exercise, individuals should start slowly, gradually increasing the difficulty level to avoid injury. Regular practice is key to seeing improvements in proprioception.

Name of the Exercise	Targeted Muscles	Repetitions Per Day
Single-Leg Stand	Glutes, Quadriceps, Hamstrings, Calves	10
BOSU Ball Squats	Quadriceps, Glutes, Core	10
Heel-to-Toe Walk	Calves, Core, Quadriceps, Glutes	10
Lateral Walks with Band	Glutes, Quadriceps, Hamstrings	10
Balance Beam Walk	Quadriceps, Glutes, Core	10
Single-Leg Deadlift	Hamstrings, Glutes, Lower back	10
Stability Ball Push-ups	Chest, Shoulders, Triceps, Core	10
Wobble Board Tilts	Calves, Quadriceps, Glutes, Core	10
Medicine Ball Catches	Shoulders, Arms, Core	10
Yoga Tree Pose	Quadriceps, Glutes, Core, Calves	10

HOW TO PERFORM THESE EXERCISES

1. Single-Leg Stand: Stand on one leg, keeping your knee slightly bent. Try to maintain your balance for a set amount of time, then switch legs.

2. BOSU Ball Squats: Stand on a BOSU ball with your feet hip-width apart. Lower your body into a squat, then rise back up to the starting position.

3. Heel-to-Toe Walk: Walk in a straight line, placing your heel directly in front of your other foot's toes with each step. Keep your arms out to your sides for balance.

4. Lateral Walks with Band: Place a resistance band around your ankles. Take steps to the side, keeping the band taut. Repeat in the opposite direction.

5. Balance Beam Walk: Walk along a balance beam or straight line, one foot directly in front of the other. Extend your arms to the side for balance.

6. Single-Leg Deadlift: Stand on one leg. With a slight bend in the standing leg, lean forward and extend your free leg behind you. Return to the starting position and switch legs.

7. Stability Ball Push-ups: With your hands on a stability ball, perform a push-up. Try to maintain your balance throughout the movement.

8. Wobble Board Tilts: Stand on a wobble board. Try to tilt the board in different directions without letting the edges touch the floor.

9. Medicine Ball Catches: Stand with your feet hip-width apart. Have a partner gently toss a medicine ball to you. Catch the ball and throw it back, maintaining your balance.

10. Yoga Tree Pose: Stand on one foot. Bend your other knee and place the sole of your foot on your inner thigh or calf (not on the knee), with toes pointing down. Bring your hands together in front of your chest, or extend them above your head.

AQUATIC THERAPY

OVERVIEW

Aquatic therapy, also known as water therapy or hydrotherapy, is a form of physical therapy that takes place in a pool or other aquatic environment. The buoyancy, resistance, and temperature of the water can help reduce the impact of movements, decrease pain, and improve circulation, making it a beneficial form of therapy for many individuals.

It's often used for rehabilitation after surgery or injury, as well as for managing chronic conditions like arthritis or fibromyalgia. The water provides a low-impact environment that reduces stress on the joints and can make movement easier for individuals with mobility issues.

Exercises in aquatic therapy can range from simple movements like walking or stretching to more complex activities like water aerobics or resistance training. The exercises can be adapted to suit individuals of different fitness levels and health conditions.

Aquatic therapy should always be carried out under the guidance of a trained professional to ensure safety and efficacy. The professional can provide individualized exercises and monitor progress to ensure the bene!ts of therapy are being realized.

Name of the Exercise	Targeted Muscles	Repetitions Per Day
Water Walking or Jogging	Legs, Core	10-15 minutes
Leg Lifts	Quadriceps, Hamstrings	10 each leg
Arm Curls	Biceps, Triceps	10 each arm
Flutter Kicking	Quadriceps, Hamstrings, Glutes	10-15 minutes
Pool Planks	Core, Shoulders	5-10
Shoulder Rolls	Shoulders, Upper Back	10 each direction
Standing Jump	Legs, Core	10
Water Push-ups	Chest, Shoulders, Arms	10
Treading Water	Whole Body	5-10 minutes
Poolside Squats	Quadriceps, Glutes, Hamstrings	10

HOW TO PERFORM THESE EXERCISES

1. Water Walking or Jogging: Walk or jog from one side of the pool to the other. Keep your back straight and use your arms for balance.

2. Leg Lifts: Stand in the pool and lift one leg to the side, then back down. Repeat with the other leg.

3. Arm Curls: With water weights, perform a bicep curl, then a tricep extension. Repeat with the other arm.

4. Flutter Kicking: Hold onto the side of the pool, stretch your body out and kick your legs.

5. Pool Planks: Use a pool noodle or foam aquatics mat. Keep your body in a straight line and hold the position.

6. Shoulder Rolls: Submerge your body up to your neck and roll your shoulders forward, then backward.

7. Standing Jump: Stand in the pool and jump as high as you can, bringing your knees into your chest.

8. Water Push-ups: Stand by the pool wall and perform a push-up motion against the wall.

9. Treading Water: Stay in one place and use your arms and legs to stay afloat.

10. Poolside Squats: Stand with your back to the pool wall, lower your body into a squat, then return to standing.

AFTERWORD

"Bending But Not Breaking: Living with Ehlers-Danlos Syndrome" by Dr. Mohammad E. Barbati is an invaluable resource for anyone seeking to understand the complexities and challenges associated with Ehlers-Danlos Syndrome (EDS) and other connective tissue disorders. It is an impressive amalgamation of detail, specificity, and empathy, offering readers both professional insight and human understanding.

From its opening pages, the book provides an in-depth exploration of EDS, a group of inherited disorders that affect the body's connective tissues, which are vital to the structure and stability of our organs, joints, and skin. The author's meticulous approach offers the reader a comprehensive understanding of these conditions, which can drastically impact an individual's quality of life.

The book's strength lies in its ability to translate complex medical concepts into a language that is accessible to a broad audience. It captures the broad spectrum of connective tissue disorders, both inherited and acquired, and offers keen insights into their unique characteristics and manifestations.

In this way, the book serves as a valuable guide for those living with these conditions, their loved ones, and healthcare professionals seeking a more profound understanding.

One of the most commendable aspects of "Bending But Not Breaking" is its exploration of the classification and subtypes of EDS. By detailing the evolution of EDS classification and the underlying genetics of the disorder, the book provides a comprehensive framework that aids in accurate diagnosis and management. This foundational knowledge is critical for the development of targeted therapies and personalized treatment plans.

While the content we have at our disposal is truncated, it's clear that the book continues to delve into the nuances of various EDS subtypes. This dedication to detail and thoroughness is a testament to the author's commitment to enhancing our understanding of these disorders.

"Bending But Not Breaking" underscores the importance of continued research and advancements in the field of connective tissue disorders. The book is not just an informational resource but also a beacon of hope for those living with conditions like EDS. It signifies a promise of better diagnostic tools, improved management strategies, and the potential for effective treatments that can improve the quality of life for those affected.

This book stands as a testament to the resilience and endurance of those living with EDS and other connective tissue disorders. It underscores the fact that, despite the challenges they face, they are 'bending but not breaking.' As we turn the final pages, we are left with a greater understanding of these conditions and a renewed sense of empathy and respect for those who navigate life with them each day.

About the Author

Dr. Mohammad E. Barbati is a consultant vascular and endovascular surgeon. He obtained an MD in endovascular treatment of venous diseases from University Hospital, Aachen. In 2018 he was appointed as a consultant vascular surgeon and lecturer at University Hospital Aachen. Dr. Barbati has been a principal or co-investigator in several clinical trials and studies involving 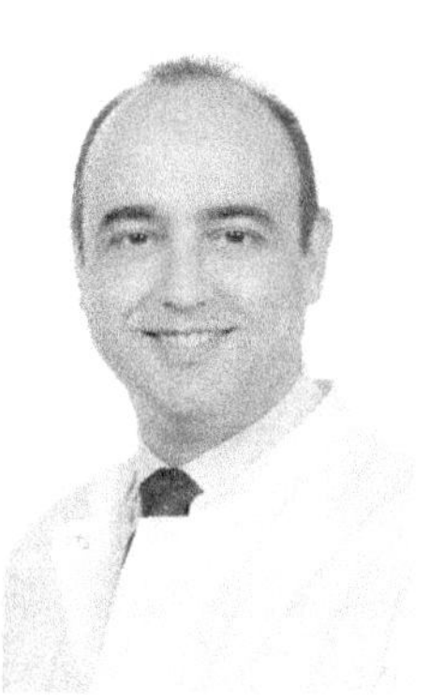 interventional treatment of DVT, PCS, PTS and other vascular diseases. To date, he has authored or co-authored more than 60 scientific publications, abstracts and book chapters. He has given over 100 invited lectures at national and international meetings and is a consultant to many medical device manufacturers.